HOW TO STRENGTHEN IMMUNITY IN 90 DAYS

Learn how to not only strengthen your immunity but also heal your digestion, hormonal, skin and autoimmune diseases with food and proper food preparation!

Nicole Lukášková

Warning:

Whenever I mention acidification in the body, I mean acidification from a holistic point of view, not from a biochemical point of view. Whenever I mention a weakness in an area of the body, I mean an energy weakness, not a physical problem in that area.

Declaration:

The text summarizes my personal experiences based on the connection of traditional treatment systems and modern research. It is intended primarily for prevention. Not a medical recommendation. I'm not a doctor. Consult your doctor for any health problems and you should also consult your doctor before making any changes to your diet. The entire material is intended for educational purposes only. It is not a substitute for treatment or medical advice.

Thank you for not distributing the Book. I offer the Book for a very low price so that everyone can afford it. By purchasing the book, you support my further work. At the same time, I would like to thank you for any recommendations to your friends and family for whom long-term health is important and they are ready for a change in their lives.

HOW TO STRENGTHEN IMMUNITY IN 90 DAYS

My holistic / comprehensive approach to health

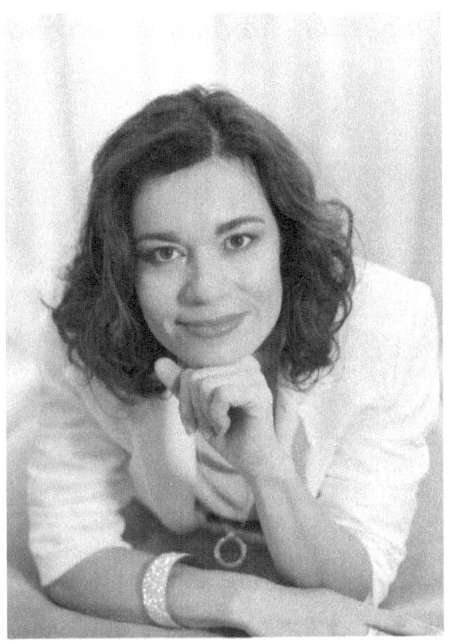

I am a holistic therapist and nutrition consultant.

I comprehensively address the **CAUSES of health problems and a preventive approach** to health. Using bioresonance, diet modification and herbs.

I adjust the diet for clients to support **the overall balance in the body** and energy-weakened areas.

Bioresonance returns the body to balance in terms of frequency, has a positive effect on the psyche and corrects entire organ pathways. Thanks to very accurate diagnostics, **this frequency therapy** eliminates loads and toxins in the body (viral, bacterial, fungi or heavy metals). The body and mind thus move towards **their own self-regulation of health**.

I test food intolerances and allergens. This method makes it possible to **eliminate burdens, solve autoimmune disorders, chronic and acute problems and hormonal imbalances**.

If interested, I work with herbs and mind relaxation techniques. This comprehensive approach is **very effective, non-invasive and without side effects**.

Nicole Lukášková, Ph.D.

HOW TO STRENGTHEN IMMUNITY IN 90 DAYS

Learn how to strengthen not only your immunity but also heal your digestion, hormonal, skin and autoimmune diseases with food and proper food preparation!

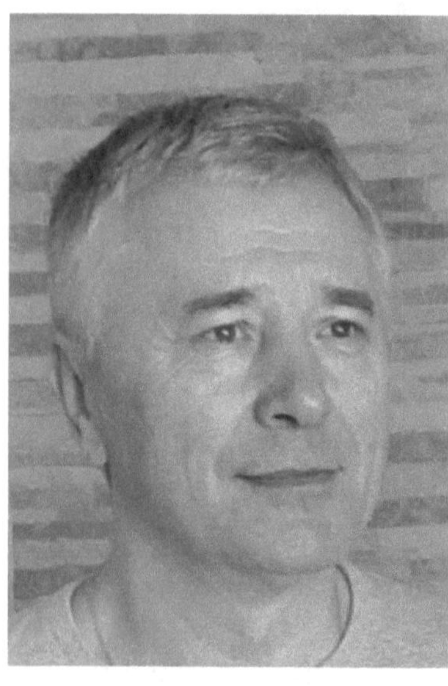

MUDr. Stanislav Rössler, a holistic physician, wrote about the Book:

"Given that a weakened immune system is the cause of a number of diseases, after reading Nicole Lukášková's e-book, I see the light in the tunnel, how in a simple way each of us can help restart our immunity. Nicole presents clear, concise, scientifically based facts, and it's up to us to follow her recommendations. I also found a number of so-called AHA moments in it, which I will try to use, especially in eating habits. I am happy to recommend the book to anyone who is not indifferent to health. "

Table of Contents

1. WHERE IS THE BASIS OF LONG-TERM IMMUNITY? 7

2. CONNECTION: IN THE BODY, EVERYTHING IS CONNECTED TO EVERYTHING 12

3. 5 STEPS TO STRENGTHENING IMMUNITY 17

4. STEP 1: REMOVE THE PATHOGENIC MICROFLORA 18

    4.1 Elimination of unsuitable foods 18

        4.1.1 Is it necessary to avoid gluten? 18

        4.1.2 Milk and milk products 21

        4.1.3 Sugar 22

        4.1.4 High processed products, preservatives 23

    4.2 Elimination of pathogens 24

5. STEP 2: STRENGTHEN DIGESTION QUALITY 26

    5.1 Anti-nutrients (antinutritional substances) in food 26

    5.2. Vegetables: its preparation for quality digestion 31

    5.3. Cereals: how to prepare them to increase their usefulness 37

    5.4. Protein - meat, fish, eggs, dairy products, legumes: how much and the right preparation 39

    5.5. Fruit: how to get the maximum for the minimum 41

    5.6. Seeds and nuts: practically indigestible when raw 41

    5.7. Sprouts: why include them in the spring 43

    5.8 Herbs and spices that support the quality of digestion 44

6. STEP 3: SUPPORT ESSENTIAL BACTERIA 46

7. STEP 4: HEAL INTESTINES 50

    7.1 Breakfast: the basis of quality of digestion (4 basic recommendations) 50

    7.2 The structure of the menu 56

    7.3 Basic recommendations on how to influence your diet through your lifestyle 62

    7.4 Heal condiments maintaining healthy digestion 65

    7.5 Suitable nutritional supplements 69

8. STEP 5: MAINTAIN A LIFE BALANCE 71

    8.1 10 simple rituals to support immunity 71

    8.2 Mind relaxation techniques 73

9. SAMPLE MENU ACCORDING TO YOUR TASTE, NEEDS AND CONDITION 78

10. SUPPORTING RECIPES 84

Vegetable alkaline broth 85

Meat bone broth 87

Winter strengthening bowl 89

Rice porridge with sweet vegetables 91

Sparse vegetable soup with miso paste 93

Congee porridge with gomasio 95

Lentil curry with rice 97

Pike perch on baked vegetables 98

Natto with rice and compressed salad 99

Trout with nishime vegetables 101

Cod baked with carrots 102

Fast vegetables with adzuki 103

Meat, fish or tempeh with nihime vegetables 104

Apple gingerbread 105

Low carb pumpkin cake 107

Sprouted chickpeas 108

Fermented buckwheat bread 110

Fermented cabbage juice 112

Healthy sweet drink 114

11. CONCLUSION 116

1. WHERE IS THE BASIS OF LONG-TERM IMMUNITY?

In addition, the year 2020 showed us how **crucial it is to build natural health and long-term immunity**. An absolutely key role for the immune system is our diet. 70% (sometimes reported up to 80%) of **the entire immune system** is concentrated in the intestinal mucosa.

The intestine is the central area where the most important processes such as nutrient absorption, energy production and the immune response take place.

If digestion does not work properly, it can also lead to the so-called leaky bowel syndrome, which can be a root problem of the following:

- **Autoimmune diseases**
- **Hormonal imbalances**
- **Asthma, eczema**
- **Inflammatory diseases**
- **Chronic fatigue**
- **Sleep disorder**
- **Depression and anxiety**

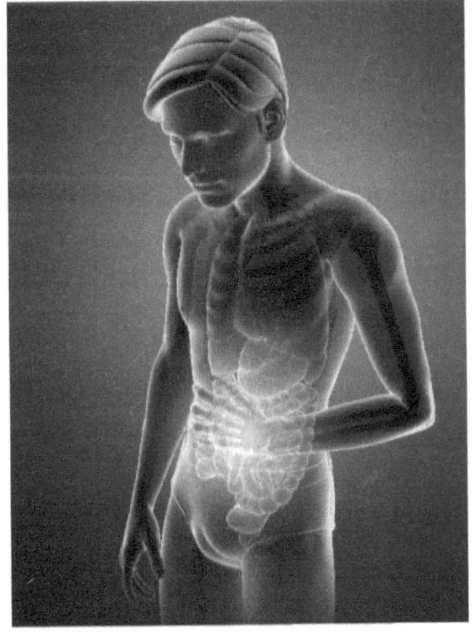

Proper digestive function is **the basis of our physical health** and, according to recent research, it is also **the basis of our mental health.**

Thanks to the fact that **we can best influence this area in the body with our diet**, the path is actually simple. We can decide every day about the quality of food, and therefore about our ability to digest and maintain a natural, healthy balance in the body. It is not enough to look at food only with an analytical view of the content of nutrients but also **how energetically it works (how it supports or worsens the quality of our digestion) in our body and how many nutrients we are able to digest from it.**

The best way to ensure good immunity is to clean your bowel. However, no drastic diet is needed. Detoxification can be done just as well with simple changes:

Firstly, the right choice of food

Secondly, its correct adjustment.

Do you want to increase non-specific immunity?

Do you want to protect yourself from the so-called diseases of civilization, or just get rid of the problems of constant coughing, runny nose and vomiting in the winter?

Then, follow these instructions. Don't be discouraged by the amount of information. I want the maximum basic context for you so that you can take responsibility for your own health. Whether you take them all at once or serve them gradually, it's up to you. Don't stress it too much! Approach yourself with love and include the joy of new changes; cleansing the body and enjoying long-term health.

Background info:

Intestinal microbiome

The so-called intestinal microbiome (our microflora), is estimated to be about 100 trillion microorganisms that inhabit our intestines. It is literally a parallel world going on in our body. The diversity of the microbiome affects the development of many so-called civilization diseases, as well as affects our behavior and psyche through the so-called gut-brain axis. All the functions of the intestinal microbiome and its effects on partial functions in the body are still the subject of research. Our diet affects the composition and diversity of the intestinal microflora, which literally "speaks" to our immune system. According to scientists, we can observe changes in the composition of the intestinal microbiome even 24 hours after a change in diet.

In a nutshell:

The intestine is the body's largest organ.

Its basic function is to release digested nutrients, while protecting against the penetration of pollutants.

The intestinal mucosa is home to many intestinal bacteria, which help to utilize nutrients. There are up to 100 trillion of them (more than cells in the body).

The mucosa is currently home to 70 to 80 % of all immune cells.

The immune system must respect the bacteria that help to utilize nutrients and at the same time fight the bacteria that try to cross the barrier of the intestinal mucosa and cause inflammation.

Regardless of research as to which microbes are beneficial to health and which are pathogenic, the most important fact for us is that **their**

diversity and balance is absolutely essential for our overall balanced health.

Area of immunity

If the gut is not in order, there is also a risk of increased leakage (so-called leaky gut). Toxins and protein molecules enter the bloodstream, causing an inflammatory environment in various parts of the body, causing autoimmune problems. A healthy intestinal environment and the balance of the intestinal microbiome is a prerequisite for a healthy immunity.

Mental health

If we do not have a healthy intestinal environment, we do not produce enough serotonin (the so-called hormone of happiness and good mood). Which in turn, is a precursor (pre-level) of melatonin, a hormone of our quality sleep. No wonder people who suffer from depression also have trouble sleeping!

Sufficient melatonin is, among other things, an essential protection against the current viral disease. In this context, we are back to the fundamental need for a healthy intestinal environment.

What causes an imbalance in the large intestine?

- Improper composition and preparation of food, fast food and semi-finished products with a large amount of added substances (dyes, flavorings, preservatives).

- Lack of fiber.
- Long-term stress.
- Some drugs - antibiotics, analgesics, cytostatics and some types of contraception.
- Smoking, alcohol, coffee (on an empty stomach).
- Lack of sleep.

2. CONNECTION: IN THE BODY, EVERYTHING IS CONNECTED TO EVERYTHING

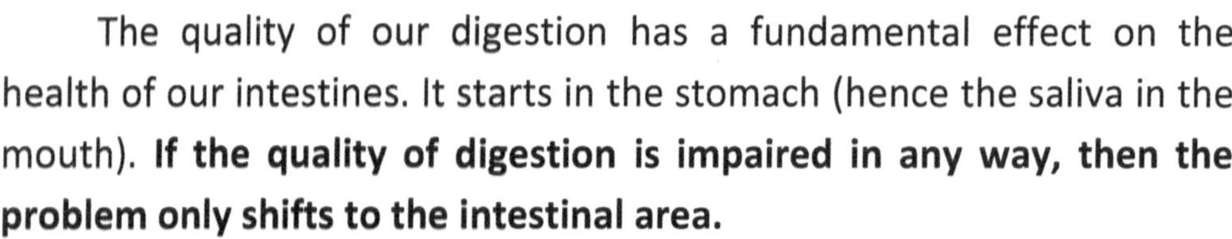

Traditional healing systems already knew that the intestine was the basis of our overall health, and modern medicine has also confirmed this by research. Our diet, stress and overall life approach determine what our immunity will be like during the winter and what the level of spring fatigue will be.

The quality of our digestion has a fundamental effect on the health of our intestines. It starts in the stomach (hence the saliva in the mouth). **If the quality of digestion is impaired in any way, then the problem only shifts to the intestinal area.**

How do I know that my digestion is weakened?

There are many symptoms, ranging from subjective signs of impaired digestion to "modern" diseases. Today, more and more people suffer from abdominal pain, flatulence, belching, **heartburn**, constipation or irritable bowel syndrome, bad breath, excessive fatigue, insufficient absorption of vitamins and minerals, yeast overgrowth, food allergies, increased intestinal permeability, **inflammation** and **autoimmune diseases**.

According to research, up to two thirds of people have some digestive problems. However, **weakened digestion** does not always have its visible symptoms. In fact, a lot of people who don't even know about it suffer from it. It is the area of digestion that is the simplest area, which we can strengthen in the best way with the right diet, every day.

I, myself struggled with chronic fatigue for many years and looked for all possible solutions. Looking back, I already knew at that time it was useless to analyze the adrenal glands and solve cortisol tests. Today, I do not have such problems. By correcting my diet, I have strengthened the quality of digestion and holistically regenerated the function of the weakened pancreas. Figuratively speaking: there is no point in solving why a hitched carriage is not going well, and not noticing that a horse is already stumbling in front.

Everything is connected in the body

Weakened digestion quality leads to cascading problems that clients do not necessarily perceive physically. Improperly digested food causes a problem in the intestinal tract. Chronic intestinal irritation leads to some subclinical inflammation, and this manifests itself in:

1) Firstly, **a change in the microbial population of the intestine**, which leads to an unhealthy intestinal environment.

2) Secondly, **disorders of nutrient absorption** (necessary for the functioning of all systems in the body).

Today, the saying, "You are what you eat.", is no longer valid. We are not what we eat, but we are what we digest. If the quality of our digestion is permanently impaired for some reason (inappropriate diet, weakened pancreas, stress, etc.), then we can eat the world's superfoods, but it is a question of how much nutritional value we are able to derive from them.

3) Lastly, **a disorder of the intestinal barrier** which is also called the **leaky gut syndrome**, (according to American estimates, it affects up to two-thirds of Americans). The disorder occurs when substances which should not be in the gut pass trough the intestinal wall. If the substances form in the gut they should also exit the gut.

It's not that we eat something and then we feel down, but it is **the basis of immune and autoimmune disorders, allergies, and various metabolic disorders**. These always have a multifactorial cause, but the impaired quality of digestion is always in their background.

Client story 1:

The client had a **reduced thyroid function** (autoimmune inflammation), she was taking Euthyrox. But over time, more and more problems with food intolerance and allergies started to appear, when she was already afraid to eat anything and use any cosmetics, which also disrupted her mental well-being. Through a holistic approach, diet modification, and frequency elimination of the loads that the body removed from its natural balance, we managed to regenerate the intestine. The client's low doses of Euthyrox remained, but she got rid of all the disease-related problems that reduced her quality of life.

Client story 2:

The client, 12 years old, **reduced thyroid function** (autoimmune inflammation). After several holistic therapies including diet modification, bowel regeneration, and thyroid gland, the girl is healthy and without medication.

Client Story 3:

Rheumatoid arthritis, female (55 years). Proper diet and quality of digestion are essential for autoimmune disorders. However, this client was not willing to adjust the menu. Nevertheless, I managed to reduce joint pain by 60% within four months of frequency therapy. We could have probably achieved even more if there was a greater degree of active cooperation in diet.

Strengthening specific areas will also improve the emotional balance

Every energy area in the body is connected to a specific emotion. Weakening of **the area / circuit of the spleen / pancreas** is associated with excessive care, memory problems, lack of concentration, fear, cumbersome thinking, distrust, etc. **The area / circuit of the intestine (and lungs) is generally associated with the emotion of sadness.** This also includes inferiority, self-pity, and depression.

I know from clients' experience that with the gradual elimination of the causes of their chronic problems in a specific area, their emotional settings also improve. They feel physical and **mental relaxation and internal emotional pressure is reduced**. In the case of the intestinal tract, it is precisely the feeling of greater joy that will be noticed by their surroundings. Of course, if by frequency we eliminate these energy pressures and specific loads in the body (eg. **fungi, bacteria, viruses, food intolerances**, etc.), people will start to feel much better mentally, emotionally, and thus experience a higher quality of life. It follows that as the weakened area is strengthened, the emotional balance associated with it is also strengthened.

3. 5 STEPS TO STRENGTHENING IMMUNITY

Here is a comprehensive and practical guide on how to strengthen immunity and health. Whether you strengthen your immunity in 90 days or in 20 days, depends on the line you are starting from. What is your current lifestyle and diet? Anyway, the positive influences and changes in how you feel physically, how your cravings change for sweets, you will recognize the change in your emotional and mental settings much earlier.

COMPLEX AND PRACTICAL GUIDE ON HOW TO:

1. **Remove pathogenic microflora**
   Elimination of unsuitable foods and elimination of pathogens

2. **Strengthen digestion quality by appropriate food preparation**

3. **Support essential bacteria**
   Fermented foods, probiotics, prebiotics

4. **Heal intestines**
   A diet that supports digestion, dietary supplements

5. **Maintain healing diet and life balance**
   Diet, exercise, relaxed mind, sleep, inner satisfaction

Each of these steps is important, but only all the steps together lead to the regeneration of the intestine, and thus to the strengthening of immunity. None of the steps 1-4 makes sense unless we include step 5. - and that is **a new lifestyle**.

4. STEP 1: REMOVE THE PATHOGENIC MICROFLORA

4.1 Elimination of unsuitable foods

You may have heard of them, but if you do not work with this information in your diet, it is the same **as if you had never heard of them**.

4.1.1 Is it necessary to avoid gluten?

If we use white flour and products made from it, then the reasons for avoiding gluten are logical. They are depleted of minerals, vitamins, enzymes and essential fiber. All that remains is gluten (cereal protein) and starch. Especially in the baked form, gluten is bound to starch, so it does not decompose in the stomach and forms a string in the intestines. These damage the intestinal wall by blocking the normal functioning of the intestinal villi, and in addition, allow the acidic environment to penetrate from the stomach into the alkaline intestine. Gluten enters the bloodstream through this damaged intestine and triggers a complex immune response.[1]

On the other hand, even whole meal bread does not have to be an overall win. If it has not been modified by the technique of our wise ancestors, i.e. by long-term fermentation (during which microbes will improve the digestibility of gluten for us), then it also contains so-called **phytates** (see chapter 5.1), which block the absorption of already population-deficient minerals such as magnesium, calcium, iron and

---

[1] Strnadelová, V., Zerzán, J., *Radost z jídla*. 6. doplněné vyd., Olomouc: Nakladatelství ANAG, 2011. 978-80-7263-704-1.

zinc. **It is important to look at each food in the context of the overall effect**.

At the same time, a simple solution (if not for celiac disease) from this pernicious modern fast food, would be a return to our roots and to a holistic / comprehensive view of health. Our ancestors ate bread, but only sparingly. They usually ate hot porridge for breakfast, which warmed them, gave them energy, and did not imaginarily cover their minds with gluten. They baked bread from whole grain and prepared it quite intuitively with a long fermentation process (naturally fermenting process without yeasts or fermentation mixtures), which reduces the amount of **phytic acid and the content of problem gluten, and improves the digestibility of bread.**

The problem, however, is that instead of returning to healthy roots and thoughtful changes in the diet, we just throw ourselves into an alternative product that does not contain gluten, but overall - from a holistic point of view - does not benefit us at all. An example of this is a quantity of gluten-free pastries with a long shelf life, containing a long list of ingredients to replace the gluing of the dough with gluten. Another deterrent example is extruded crispy slices of "bread", which are made from gluten-free cereals and thus fulfill the goal of the absence of gluten, but it is **a highly processed food with a high glycemic index and no nutritional value**. Of course, there can be no question of strengthening the quality of our digestion.

Pastries have become a modern fast food and many people cannot imagine what to actually have for breakfast and dinner. They do not know what to put ham or jam on. This has been deteriorating the intestinal mucosa for several generations. Of course, gluten is not alone in this. Overall, the composition of the diet deteriorated. Dairy products, sugar, meat and antibiotic overuse have increased. All this, together with the pastry, **leads to damage to the intestinal mucosa**. This has several consequences in the body. One of them is **a significant reduction in intestinal immunity**.

What solution do I recommend?

1. **Reduce the amount of bread.** Many people eat pastries daily for breakfast, dinner, and have pasta for lunch. Include a hot breakfast (I explain the reasons in chapter 7.1) and the correct proportions of suitably prepared food on a plate (you will find in chapter 7.2 and chapter 9).

2. **If you want to have pastries from time to time**, choose pastries from **sourdough starter (leaven)**, where the entire content of flour goes through a fermentation / fermentation process, which reduces the amount of anti-nutrients and improves digestibility. Don't be fooled in the shop by some "sourdough" pastries, to which the leaven is added only for taste, and at the same time, the flour has not been fermented.

3. **Focus on pastries made of rye or gluten-free flour.** In 10 years of my practice, I have never met anyone who would benefit from wheat. In many cases, however, gluten in general is not tolerated. With frequency therapy of the intestine and general detoxification of the body, I achieve in clients an increase in their tolerance of gluten. (Unless it is celiac disease. There is at least a significant improvement in the overall quality of life).

4. **Prepare hot dinners.** This is important not only in that you avoid pastries, but you also support the quality of digestion with a supportive diet and appropriate treatment. A warm and complete

dinner (see the structure of chapter 7.2 The structure of the menu) is especially important if we cannot indulge in a quality lunch during the working day.

4.1.2 Milk and milk products

The negatives of pasteurized milk for our digestion are already relatively well known in society. In particular, the fact that they damage the mucous membrane of the small intestine and intestinal immunity, thus increasing the susceptibility to diseases, allergies and other immune problems. Antibiotic treatment then damages the intestine, its mucosa is permeable and undigested milk proteins (as well as gluten) enter the bloodstream and cause serious to auto aggressive disorders of various organs. Another fact is that dairy products produce phlegm in the body.

Experience of many clients:

From my personal experience, the experience of clients and their children, I know that where we adjusted the diet and regenerated the intestine, we stopped being sick in the winter, respiratory problems, obstruction and frequent rhinitis disappeared.

Client story 4:

A boy, 17 years old, had long-term problems with **atopic eczema** and painful peeling of the skin on his fingers. Tried ointments and creams did not work. By adjusting the diet and frequency therapy, we increased the tolerance limit of milk and gluten, regenerated the intestine and gradually eliminated mold and heavy metals. In the photo you can see a comparison of the hands before solving the CAUSE of the problem and its healthy and soft skin after several holistic / complex therapies. In addition to milk, he can now eat all dairy products without restriction.

The photo compares before and after three holistic therapies:

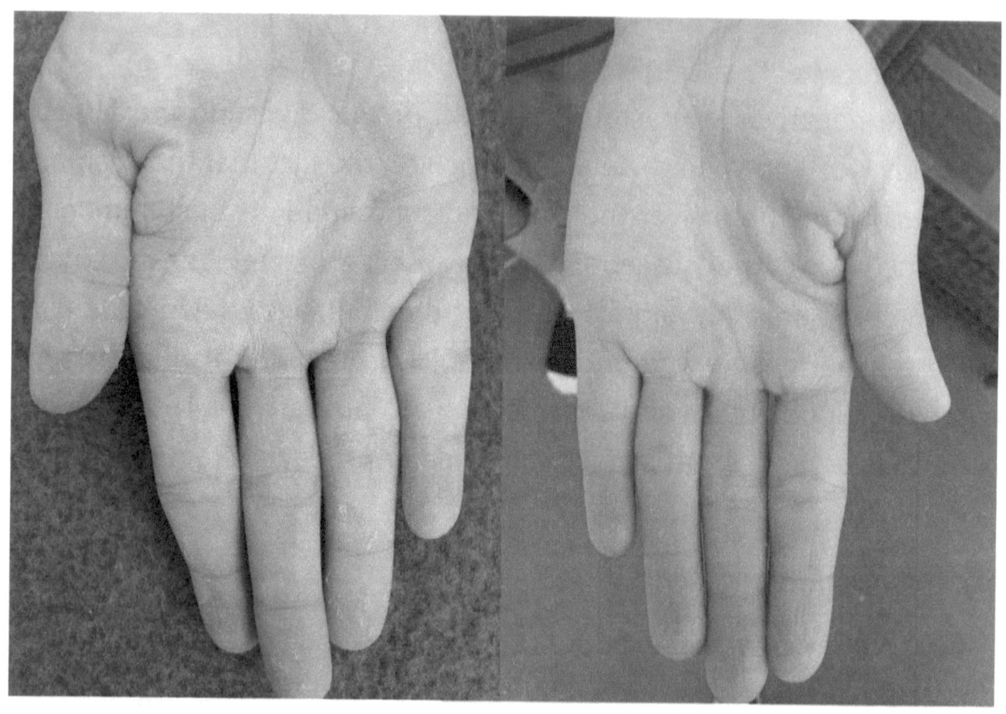

4.1.3 Sugar

Sugar is a breeding ground for fungi and parasites. The more sugar enters the gut, the faster they multiply and spread. It is not only sweet confectionery, sugary drinks but it is also part of various semi-finished and high processed products. **Sugar significantly weakens our immune system.**

Sugar is a breeding ground for fungi and their constant overgrowth disrupts not only the intestinal environment. This is not the only reason why it is necessary to exclude it from the diet. This does not mean that we will rule out a sweet taste. That would be a great pity. But we will learn how to prepare sweets from cooked fruit (see snacks in Chapter 9).

From the experience of clients, especially female clients, I know that when we eliminate mold by the frequency, they lose its irresistible sweet taste. It's not that they don't eat sweets, but they no longer have the unmanageable need to eat large amounts as in the past, and most importantly they don't have a permanent need for sweets. They can feel on **the intestine-brain axis** (see Chapter 1) that it is no longer the overgrown fungi that demand the need for sweets. They decide for themselves how much and when to eat sweets. The twelve-year-old client described it as "suddenly she did not understand her brain, why she no longer requires sweets as before."

4.1.4 High processed products, preservatives

Additives and auxiliaries such as preservatives, dyes, flavor enhancers and all man-made additives irritate and damage the intestinal wall.

- Everything canned
- Convenience food
- All highly processed foods
- Meat products - sausages, salami
- Sweetened drinks
- Sweet confectionery
- Trans Fats

- Margarines

- Artificial sweeteners, glutamates, "chemical flavors"

It's easy at first glance, but it is needed to be said here. It's all the weird food and drinks in boxes, bags and plastic bottles. You want to clean your body and not keep hurting it?

You can often hear recommendations: if you read the labels, if there is one, or a list of unknown ingredients that is too long, do not buy it. But the situation can be much simpler. You don't have to read the used ingredients at all. Basic foods such as meat, rice, millet, white yogurt or vegetables do not require a magnifying glass to read labels. Nothing else added by the food laboratory is added there.

4.2 Elimination of pathogens

Here is the key: **responsibly eliminate unsuitable food**. This way we can partially eliminate pathogens (viruses, fungi, bacteria) and not support their multiplication. In urgent cases, which are not the subject of this Book, antibiotics are, of course, necessary. Unfortunately, frequent overuse of antibiotics leads to a further imbalance of the intestinal microflora.

Furthermore, to eliminate pathogens you can use:

1. **Natural resources:**

Cleaning herbs: black cumin oil, walnut, licorice, garlic, oregano drops, thyme, cinnamon, grapefruit seed extract

Cleaning foods: Enteros gel or black coal

2. **Holistic therapy:**

This is because pathogens often persist chronically. These are mainly viruses (i.e. groups of herpes viruses, EB virus, etc.), bacteria (i.e. chronically persistent disease, chlamydia, overgrowth of coli bacteria, helicobacter pylori, etc.). Even with the chronic occurrence of these pathogens, I achieve a great effectiveness of holistic therapy in clients, which eliminates pathogens.

Another major pathogen is **overgrown internal fungi**. Fungi along with bacteria create a population in our intestines and help us complete digestion. They are a natural and necessary part of the intestinal microflora. However, the problem is that if one of the components of this system overgrows and the natural balance is disturbed, **dysbiosis occurs**. This has unfortunate consequences for our health and is the cause of many diseases that we would often not even think of in connection with the intestine. However, solving this cause is **a necessary basis for a holistic / comprehensive solution to many health problems**. Therefore, if we want to eliminate **the root CAUSE** not just treat the symptom.

Symptoms include:

- Weakened immunity

- Indigestion

- Gynecological and hormonal problems

- Skin problems

- Liver problems

- And others - all autoimmune, psychological, etc. mentioned in chap. no. 1.

The holistic therapy that I deal with then not only diagnoses these pathogens, but mainly eliminates them so that they do not cause an imbalance in the body.

Holistic therapy is based on knowledge of traditional Chinese medicine and quantum physics. It is a very effective and non-invasive method how:

- Eliminate pathogens and other loads.

- Regenerate the digestive organs and correct the entire pathways of the organs to their own function.

- Shift the body to its balance and self-regulation of health.

- Reduce emotional imbalance.

- Stabilize mentally.

5. STEP 2: STRENGTHEN DIGESTION QUALITY

Diet plays an absolutely key role in our immune system. Even though we have quality health care, we have to take responsibility for the quality of digestion ourselves. There are no drugs for that. Fortunately, we have everything in our hands and we can influence our health every day by choosing a suitable diet and the right treatment that supports digestibility.

5.1 Anti-nutrients (antinutritional substances) in food

Why is it extremely important to properly prepare foods and improve their digestibility? **Cereals, legumes, nuts and seeds** contain so-called **antinutritional substances (anti-nutrients)**, which <u>**block the absorption of nutrients and weaken our process of quality digestion.**</u>

These antinutritional substances are contained mainly in foods of plant origin and thus protect the seed or plant from predators. The content of these anti-nutrients in foods is therefore always worth reducing. We can reduce the content of these anti-nutrients by:

- **the soaking process,**

- **sprouting,**

- **fermentation (fermentation),**

- **cooking or a combination of these techniques.**

You will find these procedures for the individual foods in this chapter and also in the recipe procedure in Chapter 10.

The most important antinutritional substances that impair digestibility and block the maximum absorption of important minerals from the diet include the following:

Enzyme inhibitors - are mostly contained in cereals and legumes. These substances bind to the enzyme and thus reduce (inhibit) its activity. Therefore, it is appropriate to reduce these substances by soaking, cooking and fermentation (simple procedures are given directly in the individual recipes).

Phytic acid - is present in all plants, mostly in cereals, legumes, seeds and nuts. It tends to bind certain minerals (especially zinc, calcium, magnesium and iron) in these foods, reducing their bioavailability to the body. In other words, food contains great nutritional richness, but we must "unlock" it so that our body can reach its entire contents.

Goitrogens - are most contained in cruciferous vegetables (cabbage, broccoli, cauliflower, various types of radishes and more). These antinutritional substances complicate the metabolism of iodine, which is manifested by insufficient thyroid function. Thyroid damage can lead to excessive fatigue, overweight and irregular menstruation. Therefore, include these foods cooked or fermented instead.

Goitrogens and phytates are also contained in soy, so not only for these reasons is it not appropriate to eat other than **fermented soy products**, it is only tempeh, natto and quality soy sauce tamari or shoyu (see chapter 7.4. Flavoring healing foods). High-quality traditional soy fermentation methods neutralize anti-nutrients, improve the quality of the proteins present and increase the amount of vitamin K2, which is important, for example, for the proper use of calcium and the health of our bones.

Lectins - are primarily contained in legumes. At high doses, there is inflammation of the intestines or water retention in the lymphatic system. The content of lectins is reduced by long soaking, washing and long correct cooking (see chapter 5.4.)

Thanks to the reduction of the content of anti-nutrients, whether by soaking, germination or fermentation of food, we obtain:

1. **better digestibility**, and thus support our ability to digest food well

2. **better availability of "unlocked"** (i.e. minerals no longer blocked) minerals for the body.

As with cereals, legumes and cruciferous vegetables, it is good to reduce the content of these antinutritional substances in **nuts and larger seeds** (pumpkin, sunflower).

You can soak / activate them (at least overnight) and then use them in the morning porridge.

By activation and subsequent germination, the phytic acid content is reduced by up to two thirds. **This improves their digestibility, and "opens up" their mineral wealth to us.**

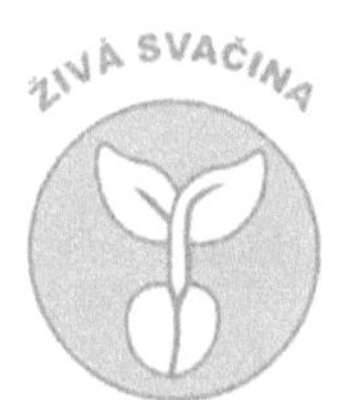

Do you want crunchy, easily digestible nuts with the maximum absorption of minerals (especially zinc, magnesium, calcium, iron), and yet you do not have time to activate them?

You can buy a sprouted nuts as a delicious, crispy snack to keep in your pocket at any time on the e-shop <u>www.ziveorechy.cz</u>

Because many people decide what to eat for snack every day, and yet the nutritional value is important to them, but they do not have time to activate and dry the nuts, in 2019 I became **the first Czech producer of activated nuts**. You can choose from several types with different "smart" flavors.

ŽIVÉ OŘECHY® activated (sprouted), yet beautifully crispy nuts gently dried to 42 ° C. *"Your snack with inner source of energy"*

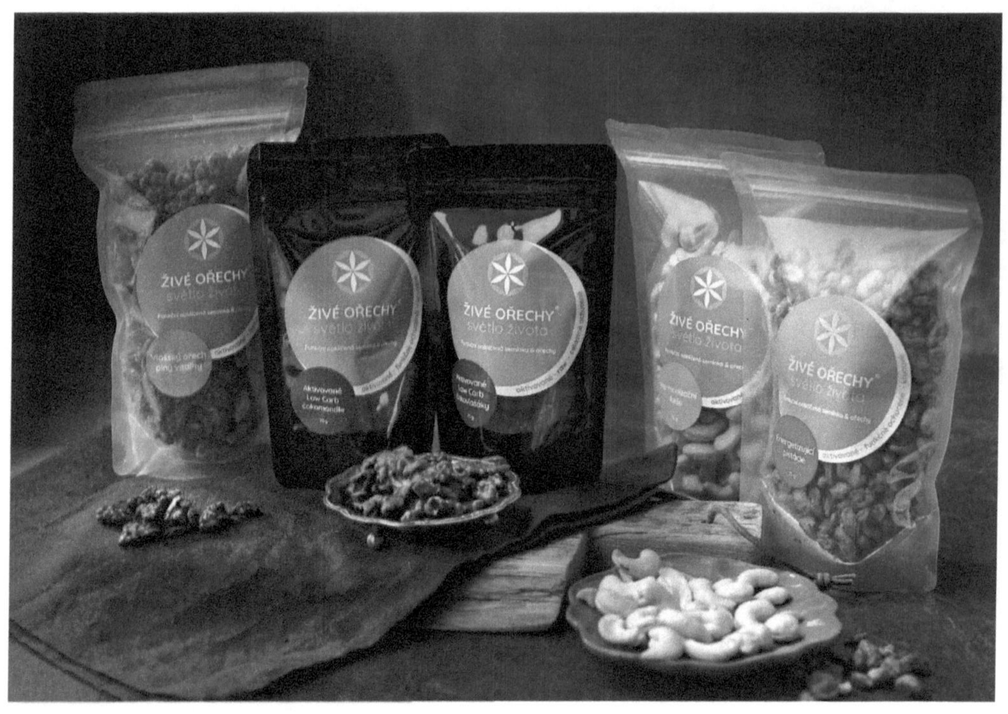

4 things you should know about ŽIVÉ OŘECHY®:

1. activated (sprouted) nuts supply the body with more available ("unlocked") minerals and are better digested,

2. are crispy, yet very finely dried to 42 ° C to remain "alive" and preserve the enzymes,

3. the whole process of their production takes up to 5 days to obtain maximum nutrients, optimal digestibility and delicate taste,

4. ŽIVÉ OŘECHY® are cleverly naturally flavored with superfoods and spices that support balance.

5.2. Vegetables: its preparation for quality digestion

Let's start with vegetables, because they are **crucial for the quality of digestion**, and therefore health in how **to adjust it properly**. I know many people **who eat a lot of vegetables and still suffer from weakened digestion**. It may seem as if their diet contains only healthy staple foods because their plates are fully lined with fresh vegetables dedicated to their health. The problem may be in the large amount of fresh vegetables (more below).

Heat-treated vegetables are much more digestible, we get more nutrients (vitamins and minerals) from them and we maintain a healthy intestinal environment for long-term immunity.

We will not dwell on the analytical view that vegetables are healthy and we need to eat them because they contain vitamins, minerals and fiber. It is important how **to adjust it so that we do not overload the digestive system and obtain maximum nutrients**. If we eat a bowl of raw salad, in addition to **loading the enzymatic functionality of the pancreas, the vegetables are under-digested and are a welcome food for mold**. In the long run, we worsen the function of the pancreas, weaken the quality of digestion, greasy stools, bloating and overgrowth of fungi.

Are you worried about the loss of vitamins by heat treatment?

Actually, the only vitamin that is reduced by heat treatment is vitamin C. However, it is already reduced by storage, so the question is how much vitamin C is in the food before it even reaches our kitchen. For some vitamins such as A, D, E, K, you increase the absorption if you prepare them together with fat. Vitamin C is supplemented over the winter with **fermented vegetables** (see Chapter 6), which has vit. C listed just one of many other positives for health.

We generally prepare vegetables for a short time, a few minutes. In summer, the preparation time is shorter than in winter. We classify frozen and dried vegetables exceptionally, rather as a supplement. **The basis should be fresh and briefly cooked vegetables**.

Of course, we also include raw vegetables to supply the vital component and enzymes. Vital energy is not storable, so a fine salad leaf will benefit you as much as its whole head. Its amount is therefore sufficient only as a supplement, which we adapt to the season. This means salads, small and big radishes **in spring and summer**. Green parsley, green onion, leek or coriander are enough for us in **the winter**. Have you seen that our grandmothers would put a plate of raw carrots, celery and parsley twice a day in the winter because they had no other vegetables? No. They ate whole cereals with warm vegetables, legumes and a spoonful of fermented vegetables and added meat on Sundays. Because it was **a way to support digestion, maintain a healthy intestinal environment and long-term immunity through diet**.

But there are more important connections that you will look for in vain in women's magazines and lifestyle portals.

Benefit No. 1: Vegetables support **the alkaline tendencies** on our plate = balances the acid-forming tendencies in the body. However, it depends on the preparation. I am talking here, of course, about fresh and short-cooked vegetables. On the contrary, once heated vegetables already have an acid-forming tendency. The same applies to any canned or sterilized vegetables. In general, the whole category of vegetables is unique, and **the only source of alkaline tendency**.

Benefit No. 2: Vegetables and fiber from it **reduce the glycemic index** (rate of increase in blood sugar).

Benefit No. 3: Fiber increases the amount of food on a plate with absolutely **minimal caloric intake**. So it works for you in the field of energy intake control.

- So eat enough vegetables of different kinds. Focus on **diversity, variability, color and freshness**. Be creative! Pick up a large basket and go around the fresh farmer market, choose what you haven't had in a long time, or be smart and economical; drive to the supermarket and buy a week supply of each type of vegetable. Then, at home, look for recipes according to your own taste, respecting the recommendations in this book, and fold your plate according to chapter 7.2 *Menu structure*. You have a plan: to **strengthen immunity and digestion quality,** if you follow the steps given here, you cannot make a mistake.
- Especially prefer heat-treated vegetables (steamed, short-boiled nishime treatment - see below), or baked in winter.

Nishime, or cooking in its own juice, is something your body will simply love. In addition, it goes well with every meal. Stack different types of vegetables (of course only one type) on the bottom of the pot, cut into larger cubes. Drizzle with water so that the vegetables do not mix (approx. 2 cm from the bottom depending on the amount of vegetables or so that they are visible without extending beyond the edge of the vegetables). Salt and cook on low heat for 10 to 20 minutes, depending on the type of vegetable and the season - longer in winter. Depending on the condition, you can add a piece of seaweed, I like the hijiki type (different types of seaweed and their importance for health can be found in chapter 7.4). To support immunity, add a slice of ginger to the bottom under the vegetables. You will find specific procedures in the recipes in chapter 10.

Steamed vegetables are especially **medicinal for the weakened, especially congested liver area**. In these cases, it is advisable to add steamed vegetables every day. The liver has many important functions, it is also an important detoxifying organ. It is not necessary to buy any steaming pots to prepare steamed vegetables. A steamer for Czech dumplings will be useful here. I still have it in the pot, ready on the stove. Put 2 cm of water on the bottom of the pot so that during cooking the steam rises into pieces of vegetables spread out on a steamer; cover with a lid and steam briefly for 2-15 minutes (leeks are really enough for a moment, while cauliflower is longer). We want vegetables for a bite, not mud. We also want good digestibility, thanks to which our body absorbs all nutrients better.

- **To enhance the quality** of digestion, use fresh vegetables on a plate only in **small quantities**. The basis is heat-treated vegetables. As you automate changes in your diet more, prepare so-called "**compressed**" salads (see below). If it doesn't work out in time, don't stress, just have a salad leaf or a piece of carrot to the main meal with warm vegetables. A small amount is enough, but it is essential.

I consider **compressed salads** to be a great invention. I would give it a Nobel Prize in the area of self-love. The owner of a weakened digestion is especially guaranteed to feel the difference from a classic salad. Suddenly no difficulty in the stomach after eating fresh salad. Lucky people with a strong "digestive fire" will realize that by preparing a compressed salad, they eat significantly more vegetables than in a normally sliced salad.

How to do it? Cut / grate the vegetables into thin slices, mix a tea/tablespoon of apple cider or umeboshi vinegar in a bowl (see chapter 7.4), press and load with a carafe of water or otherwise. Let it "work" for at least 30 minutes or a few hours. I prepare more of this salad for lunch and leave the rest of the salad under pressure to ferment at room temperature for dinner. If you have lunch away from home, you can prepare more "compressed" salad for dinner and leave the rest loaded in a glass. Be sure not to put such loaded vegetables in the refrigerator, on the contrary, leave the microbes to act at room temperature overnight. You will further support digestibility and in the morning you can take the salad with you to work as a lunch supplement.

What's the benefit? Huge:

a) Thanks to umeboshi or apple cider vinegar, vegetables become **more digestible**. Thanks to the enzymes contained in fruit vinegar (table - chemical vinegar does not contain any enzymes), vegetables are "pre-digested" and thus save our digestion. It will be easier to eat, while maintaining its fragility.

b) **Umeboshi vinegar** is a condiment with beneficial organic acids that **has the strongest alkaline tendency (reduces acidification).**

This is how we can prepare - cabbage, carrots, white radish (daikon), red radish, turnip (round white radish) or combine in various ways. For every meal, a half of cup is enough as a source of not only enzymes. We can consume it directly or we can creatively mix it with cornmeal, arugula or other fine salad.

To support immunity and new taste, you can add pressed garlic or grated horseradish to the salad. The juice of freshly grated ginger (it has **antibacterial, antiviral and anti-inflammatory effects**) is also great.

- To each main course add <u>a small amount (tablespoon)</u> of **fermented vegetables** (pickles - short-fermented vegetables, see Chapter 6 and also Recipes) to support digestion to complement a plate or part of a salad.
- Add <u>**freshly** squeezed **vegetable**</u> juice 30 minutes before the main meal. What is the benefit?
  - Additional intake of vitamins, minerals and antioxidants. If we drink the juice on an empty stomach, these nutritional micronutrients are immediately absorbed in the intestine.
  - It has **the alkaline tendency** (reduces acidification).
  - It supplies enzymes. These are essential to support digestion. According to Dr. Hiromi Shinya, M.D., an American gastroenterologist, enzymes are the key to a long and healthy life (**be careful not raw food**).
  - Thanks to the above-mentioned advantages, they are a perfect **mental and physical boost**.

It is important to drink the juice **immediately after juicing**. **Immediately** after pressing, a fast and intensive oxidation process begins, which also affects enzymes. Don't forget to **mix every sip of the juice with your saliva**. Squeeze fresh juice from **room temperature vegetables**, you do not want to cool down unnecessarily, and thus weaken the digestive area energetically.

- Prefer commonly available seasonal sources of root and above-ground vegetables. In winter it is carrots, parsley, celery, beets, pumpkins, cabbage, and brussels sprouts, leeks, in short, all the vegetables that can be commonly stored in our conditions. So avoid tomatoes during the winter.

5.3. Cereals: how to prepare them to increase their usefulness

- Discard ordinary pastries and especially classic wheat products. From your store, choose sourdough bread, not just bread where only yeast is added. The best is homemade sourdough bread, e.g. see chap. *Fermented buckwheat bread*.
- Include primarily cereals in the form of whole grains, i.e. in their natural, technologically unmodified form. Use other modified forms only for diversification.
- Gluten-free cereals - rice (alternate different types), millet, amaranth, quinoa, sorghum, buckwheat, teff.
- The whole cereals containing gluten - barley, oats, rye or kamut wheat **ferment before cooking**. How to ferment whole cereals? Let them soak overnight in water with a spoonful of apple cider or umeboshi vinegar or whey **to reduce the content of antinutritional substances** (phytic acid and enzyme blockers). You

have used the maximum amount of nutrients in these whole foods. The next day, drain the water from the cereals (there are soaked anti-nutrients), wash and cook the cereals. Fermentation doesn't cost you any extra time, it's just about planning, you have a goal: to strengthen your immunity and feel good. The **fermentation process pays off**:

- o very easy digestibility of cereals,
- o perfect saturation,
- o the amount of fiber,
- o and due to the reduction of the content of antinutrients by the fermentation process, all nutrients are "unlocked" to the body, and thus absorbable to the body.

- If the health condition allows it, choose **brown rice natural**, rather than white rice, which is "polished or cut", i.e. it is stripped of its upper skin, which contains most of the body's important vitamins (especially group B), minerals and valuable fiber. In addition, natural rice has a lower glycemic index (maintains a balanced blood sugar level) and satiates you for a longer period of time.

I like to use side dishes as a mix of two types of cereals. Thanks to this, we get both **greater variability in the diet** and in small amounts we get **a wider variability of nutrients**. For example, I cook rice together with millet, whole grains of oats, amaranth, quinoa or hatomugi.

Hatomugi also called Teardrop Barley also called Jojoba Tears is a gluten-free cereal with a shape similar to barley (you buy it in a healthy store). It has great detoxifying effects, acts in gastric and intestinal weakness and, from a holistic point of view, supports the spleen, liver, gallbladder and pancreas. Among other things, it maintains supple skin and is a great source of magnesium, calcium, zinc, potassium and iron. Just add 1/3 hatomugi to 2/3 rice and go cook.

We tell ourselves that ordinary flour and pastries from it do not benefit our digestion very much and in many cases are detrimental. If you have a quality hot breakfast and a quality dinner, then there is actually no room for pastries. Preparation will take you a little more time than getting bread or a croissant, but the difference in how you feel mentally and physically in the long run is simply **WORTH IT**. So why feed us nutritionally hungry pastries?

5.4. Protein - meat, fish, eggs, dairy products, legumes: how much and the right preparation

- If we have a sufficient amount of protein from basic foods in our diet, we will, among other things, **reduce our appetite for sweets**.
- Protein, whether of plant or animal origin, should be included in all three main meals, approximately dividing the daily amount of protein between **breakfast 20 %, lunch 45 % and dinner 35 %**. The daily intake should be about 1g of protein per 1kg of natural weight. However, there is no need to stress over mathematics and complicated calculations. A simple example is that in each main meal there should be a quantity of meat, broth from it, fish, eggs or legumes in the size of a palm. In the case of porridge, the properly prepared seeds in terms of digestibility (see chapter 5.6.).

- It is possible to combine varied and rationally different types of animal proteins (preferably farmer pastured meat, freshwater and sea wild fish, free range eggs).
- Then include various types of lentils and beans from vegetable proteins. Canned legumes are not suitable. It is best to prepare legumes in the home environment so as **to maximize their digestibility**:
    - Leave all types of legumes overnight (except for small lentils - just a few hours, red lentils, eg 15 minutes) soaked in a sufficient amount of water with a spoonful of apple cider or ume vinegar (this **will improve digestibility**),
    - Pour out the water in the morning and rinse the legumes again,
    - We cook without salt together with a pinch of satureja or marjoram and a piece of Kombu seaweed (chapter 7.4.) - spices and algae **improve the digestibility of legumes and reduce the content of anti-nutrients**. We collect the excess foam during the cooking of the legumes. We can speed up cooking in a pressure cooker, which is, among other things, also energetically suitable, especially in the cold season.
- **<u>Avoid unfermented forms of soy products</u>** (soy meat, beans, milk and other soy vegetarian products) due to the content of goitrogens, (see chap. 5.1. *Anti-nutrients*). Fermented, i.e. healthy soy products are only **tempeh, natto and quality soy sauce, such as Tamari or Shoyu.**
- Eliminate non-sour cow's dairy products. Focus on goat's and sheep's milk products, preferably in sour form again.

5.5. Fruit: how to get the maximum for the minimum

I recommend choosing from local, our geographical and seasonal sources rather than imported fruit. Exotic fruits are included in the diet only occasionally, for variety, sobriety and for medicinal reasons, such as the pomegranate superfood.

Pressed fruit juices are not suitable due to their high content of fast sugar without the presence of fiber. Prefer a smoothie or preferably whole fruit in its natural form, or slightly cooked - especially during the winter, heat-treated fruit with warming spices is suitable - cinnamon, cardamom or ginger.

If you do not eat snacks and eat only 3 times a day, I recommend chewing fruit (apple or pear) 30 minutes before lunch. **This is advantageous for several reasons**:

1. The fruit is quickly digested on an empty stomach and does not complicate the process of digestion by mixing with other foods.
2. We get enzymes from fresh fruit and thus support the process of digesting lunch.

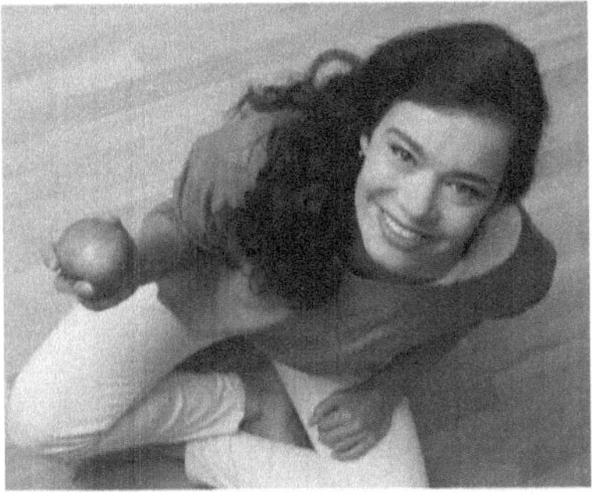

3. We are partially satisfied and then we do not rush to lunch with voracious hunger.

5.6. Seeds and nuts: practically indigestible when raw

From my practice, I see that people either do not eat nuts and seeds at all or focus more on nuts, in a form that is more burdensome for the body than beneficial. Mostly in roasted form, in large quantities and in the evening. **Nuts that are not activated are less digestible and we do not get all the nutrients we could.** In addition, their inappropriate treatment and method of consumption burdens the area of the liver, which we need to have "permeable" for both physical and emotional balance.

Of the nuts, include almonds in particular, as they are the only nuts with an alkaline tendency. Include walnuts especially in autumn and winter, they have an optimal ratio of omega-3 and omega-6 acids (simply put, the ratio of anti-inflammatory to pro-inflammatory).

As for oilseeds, they are one of the basics of the diet and it is good to include **a tablespoon in the diet every day**. Here, too, it is extremely important to properly prepare and heat-treat the seeds, as they are practically indigestible when raw. Here are the options:

a. **Roasting** - Rinse the seeds (pumpkin, sunflower or sesame) briefly in a sieve under running water. Transfer them to a hot, dry, high-bottomed pan, stir with a wide wooden spoon and sauté dry. If we would not rinse the seeds, on the one hand we would not wash away molds and desiccants, and on the other hand we would over-fry the fat in the seeds and unnecessarily put pressure on the liver.

b. **Gomasio** - is an excellent treatment of seeds with salt, which is used to salt cereals and vegetables on a plate. To make it, fry the seeds in one pan, (see previous paragraph), and dry the salt in the other pan. Crush both ingredients while still hot together in mortars. The ratio of salt and seeds is suitable 1:12 or according to the current condition. You can prepare **gomasio with sesame, pumpkin or**

flaxseed. I love black sesame especially in winter - it supports the kidney area.

c. **Cooking** - simply add the seeds to the rice and cook, cook with soup or cook in morning porridge (outmeal) or with vegetables cooked in their own juice.

- Alternate different types into your meals. These include: pumpkin seeds, sunflower, sesame, chia, flaxseed, hemp, poppy, mustard.
- With women with which we treat hormonal imbalances in a natural way, I also recommend a suitable combination of seeds in accordance with their cycle.
- Include chestnuts in autumn. **What are medicinal chestnuts medicinal in?**
    a. they support our digestion, thus supporting immunity, because immunity is not primarily about nutritional supplements but about the health of our gut and the quality of digestion,
    b. detoxifying,
    c. are suitable for rheumatism,
    d. It has a positive effect on our blood and vascular system.

I prefer to buy them hot on the street, but unfortunately this is not possible this year. So cut them and bake them in the oven yourself or add them to the cooking of porridge and cereals.

5.7. Sprouts: why include them in the spring

The sprouts are the elixir of youth, disgust and new life. They contain a large amount of vitamins, minerals and enzymes in a concentrated form. Sprouts from cruciferous vegetables (radish sprouts or broccoli) do not contain goitrogens (see chapter 5.1 Anti-nutrients). Although the germination of various seeds is extremely popular among fans of a healthy diet, you can buy sprouts in supermarkets almost all year round. Decorate your plate with fresh sprouts **primarily in the spring** (max. 1 tbsp). It is a natural period when everything in nature germinates. In terms of the so-called thermals, **the sprouts have a slightly cooling tendency**, which is something we do not need in the winter. Alternatively, we can compensate for this effect by decorating the sprouts with hot soup. You can germinate, for example, whole red or brown lentils, but you can also have sprouts of radishes, mustard, alpha, fenugreek, broccoli, etc.

5.8 Herbs and spices that support the quality of digestion

Here are herbs and spices that are good to use when cooking, making tea, or to eat with a meal. Just pour this spice into a bowl on the dining table and bite a few grains after each meal.

Spices to aid digestion and in case of indigestion:

- dill, marjoram, goodwill, thyme, cumin, saturej a or lovage, ginger, fennel, anise, coriander

Bitterness that supports digestion:

- dandelion leaves, chicory salad, dried chicory root for making tea, clove spice, black walnut, apple or wormwood

---

SUMMARY: To increase immunity in the diet is important:

- Fresh food
- Basic (technologically unprocessed) foods
- Enough fiber
- The basis is a diet with a high proportion of minerals.
- A wide range of vegetables
- Fermented foods
- Cereals - preferably whole, soaked overnight.
- Meat - best grazed, from quality sources
- Healthy fats, anti-inflammatory omega 3 acids, and conversely **reducing pro-inflammatory omega 6 acids** (they are often contained in various biscuits and confectionery, as well as in refined rape-oil and sunflower oil).
- Bone broths, soups
- Everything that has mucus protects and regenerates the intestinal mucosa - barley groats, flaxseed, chia seed, boiled long-cooked millet and rice.

6. STEP 3: SUPPORT ESSENTIAL BACTERIA

To ensure optimal intestinal balance, it is important that our diet contains so-called **probiotics**, preferably in the natural form of fermented foods. Probiotics are living microorganisms that are naturally found in the human body. Lack of probiotics in the diet can affect not only our immune system but also cause a chronic unhealthy intestinal environment and thus be the basis for autoimmune diseases.

As we said in Chapter 1, microbes in our intestines are involved in the processing of food, the functioning of immunity, affect our psyche, mood, emotions, appetite for sweets, sweetness, and therefore our weight.

So how do we best feed our intestinal microflora (microbiome)? Here is my recommendation:

Include daily:

1. **Probiotically** (living microorganisms) rich foods:
- *Fermented cabbage* (simple recipe see Recipes)
- Short fermented vegetables (pickles) - see recipe *Fermented cabbage juice*
- Lactically fermented vegetables are an excellent supplement to our diet:

  - **It strengthens the immune system and regenerates the intestine.**
  - Supports the growth of intestinal microflora.
  - Maintains a balanced composition of gastric juices.
  - Helps maintain acid-base balance (reduces acidification).

- Supports hematopoiesis

- **Tempeh** (fermented soybeans, you can buy in a health food store) - see Recipes.

- **Natto** (fermented soybeans, you can buy in a health food store) - see Recipes.

- **Miso** (see Chapter 7. 4. *Heal condiments*)

- **Kombucha** - A fermented beverage created by fermenting sweetened tea and "Tibetan mushrooms" kombucha. You can buy a drink in a healthy diet, a larger supermarket or online, or make your own - you can get kombucha on the Internet on the so-called kombucha map of sellers or donors.

- **Tibi crystals** - you will find many donors or their sellers on the Internet. Then you can propagate them yourself and donate any surpluses to your loved ones.

- For easier preparation, it is possible to buy pre-prepared dried forms, for the production of water or milk kefir.

- Include sour products such as **kefir and yogurt**. During the winter, due to the healing effect of dairy products, include these products sparingly and in the afternoon (at room temperature) rather than for breakfast, as is often "healthy" recommended (see Chapter 7).

Probiotic cultures contained in all naturally fermented foods produce lactic acid.

- **It is important for the nutrition of intestinal cells and inhibiting the growth of pathogenic bacteria.**
- **Supports the digestion of sugars and proteins.**
- **Facilitates the absorption of calcium and iron.**
- **Thus, it indirectly affects the function of the immune system.**

If, for some serious health reason, it is not possible to include probiotics in the natural diet, it is good to use them at least in capsules as a nutritional supplement.

- Probiotics are **essential for many systems** in our body.
- Add one tablespoon of fermented / fermented vegetables (**sauerkraut, kimchi or other type of fermented vegetables**) to every hot meal.
- Fermented foods give us much greater variability and complexity of beneficial bacteria than probiotics in food supplements.
- If you do not want to eat fermented vegetables and sour products (goat or sheep kefir or yogurt), buy a probiotic dietary supplement with the widest possible variety of microflora strains. Even so, I recommend supporting the intestinal microflora with a suitable fermented food supplement.

2. Prebiotic foods

Prebiotics are important in the diet because they are **food for our microbiome**. This includes all foods with fiber, especially **vegetables, properly prepared legumes and whole cereals.**

Whenever I have a lecture or a cooking workshop with children, we remind ourselves that every meal they eat should also contain the right diet (prebiotics) for the billions of animals (intestinal microflora - it is estimated that there is 1-2 kg microorganisms in our intestine). They affect our overall health, weight, sleep quality and mood.

Healthy digestion is the basis for the prevention of civilization diseases and the first, absolutely necessary step to healing.

Client story 5:

One client had huge maps of mold on 40% of the body. For half a year before she came to me, she used many antibiotics without success and tried natural options. In addition to the frequency elimination of fungi, it was necessary to eliminate the chronic presence of borreliosis, which was in the background of fungi. The basis was intestinal regeneration. Although the client did not experience any difficulties in this regard, the quality of digestion was weakened, resulting in an unhealthy intestinal environment, and thus a weakened natural immunity. **Only by eliminating these CAUSES did the CONSEQUENCES on the skin disappear.**

In this example, you can see how important the quality of our digestion is.

7. STEP 4: HEAL INTESTINES

7.1 Breakfast: the basis of quality of digestion (4 basic recommendations)

What makes breakfast essential?

Crucially, the quality and structure of breakfast affects our next diet, and our overall **physical and mental settings**. Therefore **immunity and quality of life**, also depend on this. Breakfast affects our psyche, work performance and overall balance, or, conversely, a total deviation from balance.

Stress level, blood sugar fluctuations, nutritional fullness or emptiness of breakfast all reflect performance and mental well-being.

At the same time, it does not matter what your nutritional direction is. It is important that the breakfast has certain characteristics. I call them the so-called **W.R.Z.F. breakfast**.

W.R.Z.F. breakfast

1. Warm breakfast

Breakfast should be warm to warm the center of our body and energize it. The "center" is the foundation, the pivotal point, that fulfills all the functions of digestion and metabolism. It is literally good to "melt" the fire of our digestion so that we can more effectively digest all the food we eat throughout the day. Only by sufficiently "strong" digestion do we get all the nutrients from food.

A hot breakfast starts digestion, strengthens the whole organism, and at the same time does not take away our energy. On the contrary, it supplies energy.

Best in the form of broth / thin soup with miso paste, which will give us minerals without straining. Also, in the form of porridge, preferably with vegetables, without unnecessary sugars. Cereals, especially whole grain (i.e., brown rice, oats, barley), and pseudo-cereals (i.e., millet, quinoa, amaranth) have a so-called neutral nature and do not deviate us from the **imaginary balance**. So we are not caught by any tastes, either sweet or salty. In addition, the energy is released slowly from them, so you can rest all morning, while still being mentally in your midst.

You can just have soup (I have it during the cleansing days) or just porridge, or both, one after the other. Or, you can have the soup in the morning and take the porridge with you in the thermos for a snack.

Even if you prefer a paleo or some low-carbohydrate approach, treat yourself to a cup of warm vegetable broth before breakfast. Your mineral-rich broth is very beneficial and invigorating for the digestive area.

2. Real foods

Choose primary foods without any additives and other flavorings. Thanks to breakfast made from natural ingredients, you can more easily resist over sweetened chocolate bars and highly processed meals during the day. Before you get used to a hot breakfast and if you have only had pastries for breakfast, I recommend ready-made instant mixes for beginners. But it is only a temporary recommendation. Although it is, for example, pure millet porridge without flavorings, it is technologically processed into an instant mixture, with a changed fiber structure. It has a higher glycemic index and in short: we will be hungry sooner.

3. Zero sugar

Don't overdo it or exclude so-called "healthy" sweeteners, such as honey, various sweets (cereal syrups) or fruit syrups. To strengthen immunity and health, it is better to avoid them for breakfast and rather use the basic taste of ingredients and fermentation, which promotes natural sweetness. You can then feel and know the difference after breakfast without sugar and sweeteners.

Fluctuations in blood sugar lead to mood swings, internal restlessness, hypersensitivity, fatigue and insomnia. In the long run, it leads to hyperacidity of the body, inflammation, deterioration of bones and teeth.

As for the fruit, in the morning, short-steamed fruit is significantly more digestible and invigorating for digestion than fresh fruit, on cold days with heating spices (cinnamon, cardamom, ginger). If you want to use fruit from the freezer in the morning (yes, frozen blueberries and blackberries in breakfast photos in magazines look great, but that's probably the only positive effect) and benefit your digestion, it pays to warm the fruit in this case as well. In any case, frozen foods in general are so-called "hurting" for the energy circuit of the spleen from a holistic / comprehensive point of view.

What is the treachery of sweet so-called "fitness breakfast"?

Oatmeal porridge and stacked fresh or frozen fruit are meek in the photos of magazines and Instagram accounts. They have even become an icon of a modern, healthy and fitness breakfast full of great carbohydrates that supply energy. In addition, the combination of flakes, nut butters, "healthy" sweeteners and fruit is literally a "delicacy in the mouth". You can also develop a great addiction and everyday enjoyment. **What is the treachery?**

- **The complexity of digestion** - if we have weakened digestion or take our health really seriously and want to increase immunity, we do not combine cereal porridge with fruit, syrup or any sweetener (however perceived as healthy). The reason is because **it complicates the digestion of cereals with simple sugar contained in sweeteners and fruits**. This is because this simple sugar literally shuts down the digestion of complex sugar. The whole porridge is then not thoroughly digested and becomes food for fungi that multiply. In the long run, **bloating problems can occur and fatigue can eventually come** from the initial energy and vitality. Over time, you may find that you increase portions to get enough. But in the end, you don't have to wonder how many calories you eat. Who does not believe, should try such a "fitness" diet for two weeks...

- **Higher Glycemic Index -** sweet porridge usually has a higher glycemic index and deviates us more from the imaginary center, not only due to fruit and any healthy sweeteners, but especially in the case of porridge prepared from instant mixtures. These will raise our blood sugar levels faster than porridge prepared from whole grain cereals. Overall, it is important to eat foods with a low glycemic index. After a meal with a high glycemic index, blood sugar levels rise rapidly and then fall too quickly. After a while, we have a taste for something sweet again and there will not be much of the originally planned work-productive morning. The sweet breakfast usually shows in the afternoon, when the need for something sweet returns to us like a boomerang. So, I go back to what I said at the beginning, that **breakfast affects our entire diet for the rest of the day**. With that comes our **mental performance and emotional state**.

- **Acid-forming Tendency** (from a holistic point of view) - sweet breakfast has a rather **acid-forming tendency** depending on the amount of sweeteners used. Acidification leads to fatigue and personally after such a breakfast I can hardly start a mentally productive day. Finally, even if we use "healthier" sugar alternatives, we tend to reach for something bitter that neutralizes the cravings. Unfortunately, the coffee is within easy reach.

4. Fiber

If I want **to increase immunity and maintain long-term health**, I always think about how food will affect the intestinal environment when preparing food. And is there enough food (so-called prebiotics) in my diet for the bacteria I want to support? **Prebiotics are an indigestible component of food that supports the growth or activity of the intestinal microflora and thus improves our health and immunity**. It is mainly a fiber contained primarily in cereals and vegetables.

Client experiences:

All clients who included breakfast as recommended in the holistic frequency therapy experienced the following changes: they felt better during the day, had no appetite for sweets and coffee, and were mentally focused. Particularly in women, the problems associated with hypoglycemia and estrogen dominance have improved.

Answers to questions you may have on the topic of breakfast:

? Do you get up early for work and don't think about breakfast?

- If you wake up really early in the morning, I recommend pure vegetable broth (see Recipes), which you just heat with a little miso paste or thin soup with miso paste (see Recipes and chap.7.4). Vegetable broth has huge benefits for the quality of digestion:
  - It warms and **energetically strengthens the digestive** area.
  - You supply the body with **minerals**.
  - It is **alkaline** (from a holistic point of view it reduces acidification).
- If you don't have to wake up to an alarm clock in the early morning hours and you're still not hungry, it means a learned habit or dinner was hearty or late and you just don't feel natural hunger after a night of fasting. Of course, our lifestyle and body needs are also reflected in our diet.

? Do you occasionally include intermittent fasting, so do you skip breakfast?

- Pure vegetable broth or, on the contrary, a strong broth from root vegetables will only **support your targeted detoxification**, and in addition, by heating our "center" (stomach and spleen) it will strengthen this area, "ground" and reduce the level of stress.

Note: In case of hormonal imbalance, ALWAYS eat a full breakfast with enough protein, whole cereals and vegetables to ensure a balanced blood sugar level.

? What if I don't have time to cook in the morning?

It's really not complicated and it just needs **a plan**. None of the recommended breakfasts will take you more than 10 minutes. I will advise you on tweaks to manage everything without stress.

- Meat bone broth is "made" by itself, put in a pot in the evening and done in the morning (see Recipes)
- I like to prepare fresh porridge, put it in the rice cooker and before I return from a walk with my four-legged friend, the porridge is ready on its own. Another option is to cook more side dishes (rice or millet) the day before, and in the morning just boil them with water or vegetable milk. For "beginners", I recommend to start with an instant mixture (watch only their ingredients) and an electric kettle. When you cook porridge from real millet in the weekend, you will find out how significantly different you feel compared to instant porridge. And not just after breakfast but all morning.
- You can prepare the vegetables in a closed box in the evening and let them cook briefly in the morning before preparing to leave the house.

7.2 The structure of the menu

Immediately after waking up, drink a glass of warm water with a spoonful (or according to taste) of apple cider or umeboshi vinegar (for its benefits, see chapter 7.4).
Go outside or open the window and breathe deeply (see chapter 8), stretch in your own way.

Menu structure:

Breakfast in general:
palm-sized proteins, vegetables (briefly cooked in winter),
gluten - free cereal

E.g.:
- Meat bone broth with freshly cooked vegetables and green sprinkles
- Salted porridge, vegetables, seeds
- Millet porridge with fruit and seeds, without sweeteners

60 minutes before lunch drink a large glass (300 ml) of water (warm in winter)

30 minutes before lunch chew a fresh room temperature fruit thoroughly

Simple approximate structure of lunch:

¼ plates is a food containing protein, ¼ plates are cereals, ½ plates are vegetables (of which 80% are heat-treated and 20% are compressed salad) + 1 tablespoon of fermented vegetables.

60 minutes before dinner drink a large glass (300 ml) of water (warm in winter)

30 min before dinner drink 200ml freshly squeezed <u>vegetable</u> juices, e.g. beets, carrots, celery, ginger (use room temperature vegetables)

Simple dinner structure:
A) complex dinner with the same structure as lunch:
¼ plates is a food containing protein, ¼ plates are cereals, ½ plates are vegetables (of which 80 % are heat-treated and 20 % are compressed salad) + 1 tablespoon of fermented vegetables.

B) If you prefer a low-carb dinner, substitute the side dish in favor of vegetables:
¼ plates are food with protein content, ¾ plates are vegetables (of which 80 % heat-treated and 20 % compressed salad or a piece of vegetables) + 1 tablespoon of fermented vegetables.

Include spices to aid digestion:

Ginger, fennel, anise, coriander, cumin, marjoram

Recipe for antiviral garlic water:

In the evening, prepare water (preferably filtered) in a large glass bottle or porcelain teapot and put one peeled and longitudinally cut clove of garlic in it. In the morning you have a natural antiviral drug ready.

*If you drink garlic water on an empty stomach, which is essential, garlic essential oils get directly and immediately into the small intestine, where they have **antiviral and antibacterial effects.***

Warning: use garlic water as a natural antiviral only for a limited time. Do not use it in healthy conditions where it is not appropriate to include garlic. One also needs variety. What is medicine for one can be poison for another.

Answers to questions you may have about the menu:

? Why do I not recommend water with lemon juice in the morning like everywhere in Internet?

Lemon has a markedly cooling thermal tendency. Since we need to warm our digestion in the morning, lemon is the last thing we need in the morning. The original promoters of lemon water were probably living in L.A. they had a good idea, but they don't live in as cold a zone as we do. And the Internet has spread this as a general practice. Enjoy lemon water in the morning in spring and summer. On cold days, however, **warm water with lemon is a great afternoon drink instead of coffee**. It will perfectly "boost" you, support the adrenal glands and supply vitamin C, which **is essential for immunity**.

? Where did the snacks go?

If possible, eat 3 times a day, it will benefit not only the intestines but also your weight and digestion will gain time to regenerate. **Stop snacking all the time** - it is difficult for the intestines, when with every small bite we eat we have to start the whole orchestra of digestion.

If for some reason you really need snacks, I recommend my activated (sprouted) nuts <u>ŽIVÉ OŘECHY</u>®. Because activated nuts were not available in the Czech Republic, I became their first Czech producer. I make these cleverly flavored activated (sprouted) nuts just for the need for quality snacks. It is a tasty snack for anyone who wants to eat properly. For everyone for whom nutritional value is important and if you do not have time to activate nuts and functionally flavoring them.

They are activated, i.e. soaked for a long time, to reduce the content of antinutritional substances (phytic acid and enzyme blockers) and dried to 42 ° C to be crispy, while maintaining raw quality and enzymes. Thanks to:

- They have a higher content of minerals available for the body (especially magnesium, calcium, zinc and iron),

- They are better digested,

- Their own enzymes save our digestive enzymes,

- In addition, they are cleverly naturally flavored (e.g., anti-inflammatory turmeric, stimulating quarana, or promoting a good mood with sugar from unroasted, sugar-free cocoa beans).

? What if I need a bigger snack? **I have types for you:**

If it is not possible to have dinner in time, prepare a larger snack. E.g. to nuts and seeds add:

- a warm apple or pear (either just steam or sauté with cinnamon or cardamom). Don't have time? chew a fresh room temperature fruit thoroughly.

- Take room temperature goat kefir with you to work, add a teaspoon of cocoa from unroasted cocoa beans and just shake. Why? This will tune your snack to the food of the gods, literally **full of antioxidants and magnesium**, and naturally encourage endorphins.

- Or shake the kefir with the matcha powder. Why? You will boost your mental and physical potential to heights from which you will not crash like after coffee. In addition, it will move this snack in a more **alkaline direction**.

? Do you need an even richer snack for any reason?

- When you prepare porridge in the morning, do more of it and take it to work in a thermos.
- Alternatively, you can find a simple buckwheat bread that every child can handle (you find it in the recipe section).

7.3 Basic recommendations on how to influence your diet through your lifestyle

1. Conscious consumption

Set aside space to enjoy your breakfast in peace. The mood and energy you eat breakfast will affect the overall energy of your day. In addition, you will be grateful for the food, have respect for the person who prepared the breakfast and, last but not least, have respect for yourself. According to Ayurveda, **the condition in which we eat food is much more important than the quality of the food we eat**. If we are not conscious, it is literally as if we are swallowing stress and sending acidity directly to the area of digestion. In the language of modern Western dietetics - food eaten under **stress triggers a chain reaction, which is associated with a decrease in the production of hydrochloric acid** (HCl). Its deficiency causes poor digestion, insufficient absorption of nutrients from any quality and varied diet, food intolerance and cascading health problems.

2. Chew

The process of digestion begins in the mouth. If we eliminate this step by insufficient chewing, and thus pre-digestion, we will burden the next stages of digestion. It doesn't matter if you count the number of bites or which technique of conscious biting you choose. The point is that the food is perfectly comminuted and best sintered into a liquid slurry before being swallowed. The best way to master this method of chewing is with a porridge of whole cooked grain. In addition, you will enjoy the naturally sweet taste of the complete grain. It has its advantages:

Why is it important to chew?

1. You don't eat a pile then. The brain has room to tell you in time that it is saturated.

2. Only in our mouths do we have the enzyme ptyalin, which helps us to digest our diet, especially carbohydrates. This way, we do not unnecessarily deplete valuable digestive enzymes on the next digestive pathway.

3. Saliva is alkaline. By careful chewing, we prepare even lower-quality food for digestion at a less catastrophic level.

Eat slowly. After each bite, place the cutlery on a plate. Only after you carefully chew and swallow, pick up your cutlery to prepare another bite. Eat in peace. Eat when sitting.

3. Eat your last meal at 6 p.m.

The rule of dinner before 6 pm is essential if we set our overall biorhythm (if we do not work night shifts) **to promote natural health.** This means that if we go (we should) to bed at 10 pm and get up at 6 am, then the last meal at 6 pm is completely natural and it is not logical to let the whole digestion process start again with another evening meal. On the contrary, it is very beneficial to give digestion space for regeneration, and to use quality sleep.

If food is eaten later, our body no longer has the opportunity to digest well. Then we strain it unnecessarily by spending the night digesting instead of regenerating at this time as we rest.

4. Go to bed no later than 10 pm

Good and regular sleep respecting the overall biorhythm is absolutely essential. **Irregular, too short or too long sleep increases the long-term level of stress cortisol - it blocks the immune system.**

5. Push yourself

Push yourself and eat "right" for at least 3 days in a row. It's the same as fasting. For the first three days the body used to and dependent on various stimulants in the form of sugar, coffee and chemicals in processed food products and fast foods will protest. Yeast and overpopulated hostile bacteria in the gut will claim theirs. This inner struggle of "who from whom" can flare up, whether in the form of appetite or withdrawal symptoms such as headaches (depending on the current lifestyle). In order to make the best of this, I recommend, if possible, to include a cleansing breakfast every other day only in the form of thin broths with vegetables (see *Sample Menu*, Chapter 9). See how you feel after such a diet, which is not a diet at all but a natural diet of our ancestors. Give yourself space to realize how you feel physically and mentally. It will be a great support for you to continue.

7.4 Heal condiments maintaining healthy digestion

You can buy them in most health food stores, online stores, but also larger supermarkets.

Vinegar as a support for digestion

Purely, natural vinegar obtained by fermenting fruit into wine and subsequent fermentation into vinegar (eg. apple cider or wine), is suitable as an aperitif and at the same time as a digestion aid. The sour taste is refreshing and natural vinegars, like fermented vegetables, are good for our liver. In the area of a holistic approach to health and diet, drinking water with natural vinegar or lemon is mainly a support of the so-called acid-base balance (balancing the acid-forming and alkaline action of food). Although these flavors are sour in taste, they have an alkaline effect on the body. They reduce the state of hyperacidity in the body - I mean hyperacidity from a holistic point of view, not from a biochemical point of view. Of course, it always depends on the current health condition.

Natural vinegars are suitable for dressings, sauces or just diluted with water as an aperitif before meals. Diluted vinegar therefore makes sense to drink, for example, before breakfast or before dinner. On the contrary, don't drink diluted vinegar in the evening because it is appropriate to give the digestion the time to rest. In some cultures, a carafe of water and a bottle of natural vinegar is a natural part of every table in restaurants. There are also vinegars from fermented vegetables or rice vinegars.

Personally, I like to use **umeboshi vinegar**. It has a highly alkaline effect, contains enzymes and is suitable for flavoring food at the very end, when the food is no longer cooked. Its healing effects:

- in any state of **weakened digestion,**

- acts as **a great boost,**

- and **removes the feeling of fatigue.**

Umeboshi plums - their fermentation produces the aforementioned umeboshi vinegar. They have the same healing effects as ume vinegar, of which I would underline the immediate **help with any digestive problems of various causes.**

Miso paste and its harmonizing and healing effects

Miso paste is a great ingredient for maintaining balance, and therefore natural immunity, and I add it to any soup where appropriate. It is a Japanese means of longevity and traditionally a cup of miso soup is drunk every morning and before each main meal.

Beneficial effects of miso paste:

- Traditional unpasteurized miso is a rich source of enzymes, supports digestion, and contains a large amount of minerals.

- It stimulates vitality, improves blood quality - it is beneficial for anemia, **insufficient blood supply to the limbs, cold limb syndrome,** perfectly **compensates for low blood pressure**.

- Supports healthy heart function.

- It has the ability to bind radioactive substances, heavy metals and neutralizes the effects of a polluted environment.

It is produced by fermentation. Choose a quality, unpasteurized miso. Miso is used at the end of cooking, food should no longer be cooked, just lightly dragged. We just let it happen, and for the last 2 minutes we allow the tastes to come together. We don't have to use that much salt anymore, because it was used in the fermentation production process.

Fermented soy sauce

I recommend a kind of tamari or shoyu. It is released during the maturation of dark miso soybean paste and contains a large amount of easily digestible nutrients. You will find a large number of products on the market under the name "soy sauce". Most are industrially produced without a fermentation process, contain sodium glutamate and a dark dye. If you want to support your health with food, I recommend sticking to shoyu sauce (made from soy, wheat and salt - fermentation decomposes wheat protein), which has a rich aroma and is a suitable flavor for a normal day. Tamari sauce (made by fermentation only from soybeans and salt, i.e. gluten-free), which is more expensive, thicker and more mature.

Algae,algae,algae

They are an amazing, mineral-packed supplement to harmonize our health. We ideally balance our current, mineral-poor diet (i.e. iron, calcium, potassium, but also trace elements, which is necessary for some systems in the body, but essential). They contain a component of more minerals than our common vegetables, which therefore has a major impact, is the prevention of osteoporosis and a resource that is insufficient in our conditions. They support healthy hair, nails and weight loss.

Algae were not just part of the diet in marine areas. Even outside the oceans, people consumed algae from lakes and rivers. Today, we buy nutritional supplements from these freshwater algae.

We add **wakame seaweed** to the morning soups. It softens quickly, partially dissolves. Along with algae **hijiki** and **arame** contains the most calcium. In contrast, the **kombu** and **arame** algae also contain the most iodine of all algae. If you suffer from anemia, include dulse seaweed. For starters, you can try any kind of cheaper seaweed. For example, nori in the form of flakes or a piece of slice for making sushi. A small amount about the size of a postage stamp is added to cooking (see *recipes*).

Kuzu root

Another medicinal food with holistic effects is kuzu root. It is a ground root in the form of starch, which I use for thickening and glazing, but its therapeutic use is essential:

- promotes **detoxification and strengthens** the immune system,
- strengthens the circuit of our digestion, helps with intestinal problems,
- strengthens **the nervous system**,
- increases **serotonin and dopamine levels**,
- reduces gastric hyperacidity.

7.5 Suitable nutritional supplements

It is best for our body to get micronutrients (vitamins, minerals and amino acids) from the diet. In such a form, they are in the most absorbable form, and in addition act synergistically in the body. However, there are situations, such as the current health condition or, for example, the seasons causing vitamin D deficiency in the general population, when the use of nutritional supplements is appropriate.

	Their effects
Vit. C	Essential for our immunity. If you decide to take vit. C even as a vitamin supplement, drink it with water and fresh lemon juice.
Vit. D3	• It contributes to the normal function of the immune system and the proper response to inflammatory processes. • Helps maintain the normal condition of bones and teeth.
Zinc	Necessary for the production of white blood cells (immune cells).
Vit. B group	They are essential for the healthy functioning of the metabolism.
Selenium	It acts synergistically with zinc and supports immunity.
Vit. K2	• It helps maintain the normal condition of the bones. • Supports normal heart function. • It helps maintain the normal state of the vascular system.
Omega-3	• They have an anti-inflammatory effect. • They help maintain the body's normal defenses. • They support the normal development of the brain

	and nervous system. • They support normal calcium metabolism. They help maintain normal joint mobility. • They help maintain normal blood pressure and normal levels of cholesterol and triglycerides in the blood. • They help maintain normal heart and blood vessel function. • They support the normal course of the menstrual cycle and menopause.
Vit. A	Bioactive Beta-carotene is suitable.

Vitamins A, D3 and K2 are fat-soluble vitamins. Therefore, always take them with food.

Another suitable supplement is **goat colostrum**. It is obtained from goats no later than 12 hours after the birth of their young, after the young are sufficiently fed. Thus, surplus colostrum is used. Its effects on health are:

- Significantly strengthens the immune system and supports the defense system.

- Overall, it strengthens the body and accelerates regeneration after illness or heavy stress.

8. STEP 5: MAINTAIN A LIFE BALANCE

8.1 10 simple rituals to support immunity

Why is it important to have your morning rituals? Because if we don't have our morning procedures, you can easily skip your intention and leave it for the next day and maybe until the next week. When you focus on your body and mind during your morning ritual, you enter a new day with a clear intention - **to strengthen immunity and feel good**. Here are my rituals:

1. I still feel **grateful** in bed after waking up. For what? For the next day you got here, for the opportunity to experience it differently, for the opportunity to make changes for the better in life, because no one promised us tomorrow.

2. Drink a glass of warm water with a teaspoon of umeboshi vinegar (alternatively apple cider vinegar).

3. Go outside, onto the terrace or just lean out of the window and take a deep breath several times through your nose and slowly exhale all the air through your mouth until the ribs are contracted. Add body stretching with active conscious breathing. Rather than a breathing technique, it is **a process to enhance overall energy and vitality**. Try my technique:

First, inhale freely in the abdomen and exhale completely. With a breath in your stomach, wake up with your fingers outstretched, and with a sharp exhale, pull your arms toward your body and squeeze your hands hard into your fist. The movement is sharp and the abdominal cavity moves outwards and inwards. For beginners, just do it 10 times. Then hold your breath for about 3-5 seconds and a long maximum exhalation through your nose. You can alternate weighting, preloading, and tightening. Mentally, you concentrate strength and vitality within a new day.

Complex health effects of this technique:

- stimulates digestion,

- supports intestinal peristalsis,

- **regenerates the body and improves memory,**

- strengthens the abdominal muscles and helps remove excess fat in this area,

- calms the nervous system,

- increases vitality and desire to live fully.

(This breathing exercise is not suitable for cardiac patients with pressure problems or ear pain, so feel your body's signals.)

4. Set aside time for a quality breakfast. It is a time period of the energy circuit of the stomach and spleen and it is associated with **balance, self-worth and self-love**. What we eat and how is a reflection of our relationship with each other. So if you want to strengthen this area, take care of yourself.

5. Eat every meal consciously and chew enough.

6. After 6 pm, turn off the blue light - it disrupts the body's natural biorhythm.

7. Turn off wifi and phones for the night (or set the plane mode).

8. Go to bed no later than 10 pm. If you do not have perfect darkness in the bedroom, put blackout curtains on the windows.

Respect the natural rhythm of the body for the necessary renewal and regeneration of all bodily and mental functions. Our ancestors had this knowledge many thousands of years ago. With a very perfect, yet simple method of observation, they knew at what time the individual organs in our body needed to rest and when their highest activity was the so-called **organ clock**. Modern research has already verified this knowledge, and in 2017 the Nobel Prize was awarded for the discovery of circadian rhythms.

9. Walk **at least 5 km every day**. Only another physical activity (above the 10,000 steps as a minimum natural basis) is a sporting movement.

Harden yourself. The cold constricts the lymphatic vessels and thus promotes lymphatic activity and detoxification, which is an impulse for the immune system. Take advantage of the perfection of our breath and try Yima Hof's yoga breathing here or download his application and include it in your daily routine (if your health condition allows it). It is a technique that has been shown **to reduce the inflammatory environment in the body and strengthen immunity.**

10. **Be present and feel** how you feel better physically and mentally.

8.2 Mind relaxation techniques

Long-term stress, which causes long-term elevated levels of the stress hormone cortisol, disrupts the nervous system, the hormonal system, increases inflammation in the body, and **blocks the immune system**.

Conscious breathing technique

1. Lie on your back and bend your legs at the knees. The feet touch the mat freely. Lift your head slightly and put it back on to feel that the cervical spine is flush with the whole spine. Close your eyes.
2. Place your palms on your abdomen and inhale through your nose into your abdomen so that you can feel the abdomen inflate under your hands.
3. When you feel the need to exhale, exhale slowly through your nose, and as long as your entire abdomen is empty and as if you want to "squeeze" your entire chest to maximize the capacity of your lungs.
4. Continue with normal nasal breaths and maximally prolonged nasal exhalations.
5. Try to inhale for 3 seconds, hold your breath for 4 seconds and exhale for 5 seconds. You may be able to extend your exhalation for significantly more seconds, such as 8-10 seconds. It depends on your condition and length of practice. (I mean weeks and months).

   Try Rhythm 4-7-8:

   a. Inhale through your nose for 4 seconds.
   b. Hold your breath for 7 seconds.
   c. Exhale slowly through your nose or mouth (whichever is more pleasant) for 8 seconds.
   d. Repeat the rhythm until you feel relaxed.
6. With each exhalation, visualize how, together with the air, everything insignificant and no longer functional in your life **leaves the body**. You can see the release of these things, patterns

or emotions with your inner vision or hear/feel them release. It depends on whether you are more visual, auditory or kinesthetic when relaxing.

7. Don't overdo it with the number of inhales and exhales. In the beginning, you may only need a few. Feel your body. If you get a headache, stop and next time do just enough to feel comfortable and perceive the activation, while relaxing in the abdomen and your center.

The technique of relaxing the mind through focused attention

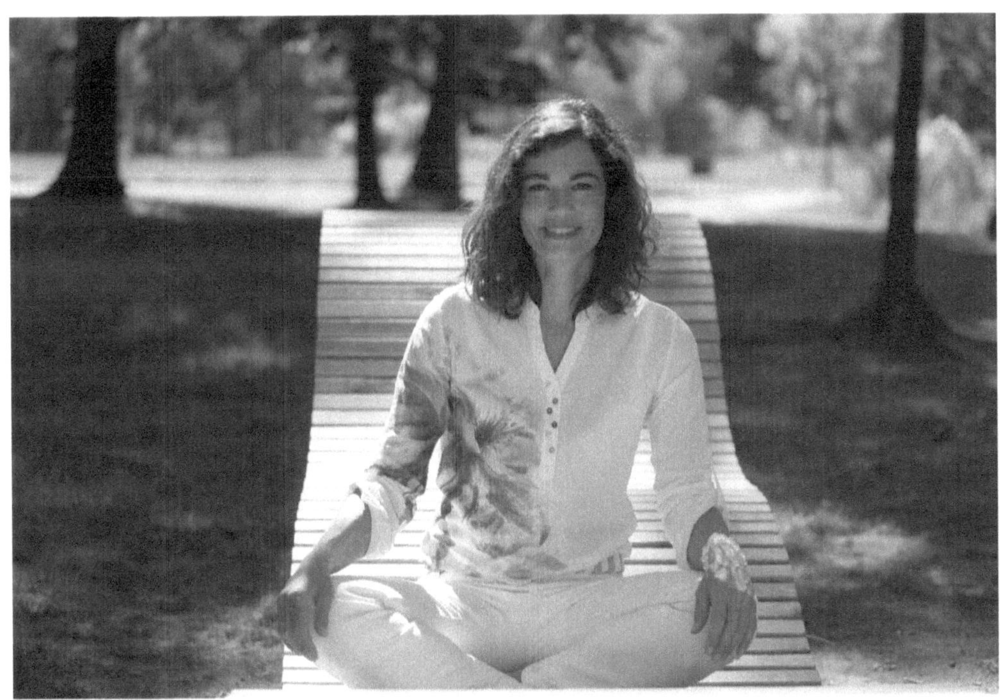

1. **Take a relaxed position** with an upright but not convulsively upright spine, lift your shoulders for a moment and let them drop freely, loosening your neck a little, your hands resting on your thighs palms down, and if you feel drowsy, insert the back of one hand into the other.
2. The lips do not press strongly together, they are relaxed, you release the tension so that the mouth is slightly open, **we place the tongue on the upper floor**.
3. We inhale and exhale several times, inhale through the nose and exhale emotionally with the feet.

Attention is focused on our nostrils, we realize how we breathe, we feel the air coming through the nostrils and leaving again. We do not analyze anything, just simple awareness. We do not follow the breath as it passes into the lungs, we do not follow its path, we focus only on the nostrils. When our attention deviates and wanders, for example, with a memory, thought or fantasy, we return our attention back to the nostrils. Nothing happens, calm and without remorse. Inhale and exhale. Inhale and exhale.

All mental functions also begin to calm down and slow down, along with the breath and thus the brainwaves. We begin to feel much calmer and more relaxed and more open, gradually ceasing to identify with the slander of the inner voice.

This is, of course, preceded by a struggle with our scattered attention and the development of simple attention, which is a simple realization of bare facts without any reaction or commentary. In everyday life (at the level of BETA consciousness) this silence of the mind is practically non-existent.

Focus your attention only on the natural perfection of the breath. It connects us to our body. With the first breath, our life begins here and with the exhalation it ends.

In mind relaxation courses, clients sometimes tell me how difficult it is to ignore incoming thoughts. It's just about practicing. You didn't even start walking right away, but you tried again and again. It's worth it. With one breath, the clients add how wonderful the calming of the mind and the relaxation of the body comes with this technique.

9. SAMPLE MENU ACCORDING TO YOUR TASTE, NEEDS AND CONDITION

The diet is designed to **maximally support the quality of digestion, intestinal health and our immunity**.

There is always soup at the main courses. Its benefit is big and perhaps in all traditional healing systems **soups are used as medicine**. If the soup is made of suitable foods and properly prepared, **it warms our center, strengthens digestion, supports the balance of the intestines, supplies minerals and has an alkaline tendency**. All this <u>contributes to the natural, and especially long-term immunity</u>. According to some research, **it also reduces the caloric requirement of the main meal**. However, if you do not manage soups for the main course, even if they are quick (see recipes), nothing happens, including only what you can handle and keep a smile on your face.

You can find the recipes in the recipe section. You can change them in any way with different types of vegetables, side dishes and types of protein (fish, legumes, meat).

Sometimes you can only include a thin soup with miso paste for a cleansing day for breakfast. Or you can have a bigger breakfast after it according to your needs and health condition.

If you do not live by active movement, reduce the number of side dishes for dinner or eliminate them completely in favor of warm vegetables.

Use your imagination and with the knowledge of everything I have said on the topic of **How to strengthen immunity in 90 days**, prepare your food according to your health and your abilities. You will find some dishes in the recipe section, according to which you can easily and variably prepare any other with variations.

Here are sample examples: (most can be found in the Recipe section)

Breakfast:

During intermittent fasting:

- Healthy sweet drink

For cleansing days or as part of a larger breakfast:

- Vegetable broth with miso paste

- Meat bone broth only with parsley, chives or coriander

- Winter toning bowl

- Sparse vegetable soup with miso paste

For cleansing days:

- Rice porridge with sweet vegetables and seeds or any cereal porridge with vegetables and seeds
- Millet porridge with chestnuts and plum broth

Therapeutic breakfast in case of great weakness, eg irritating colon:

- Porridge congee

60 min before lunch: big glass of hot water

30 min before lunch:

- Thoroughly chewed seasonal and local fruits - such as apples, pears, plums
- or pomegranate (although it is not a local fruit, I sometimes classify it for medicinal effects)

Lunch - soup:

- A mug of broth made of meat bones, if you've been left in the fridge since the last long-drawn broth
- Vegetable soup with miso paste
- Creamy vegetable soup, just from vegetable with miso paste

Lunch - main course: (combine different types of meat, legumes or fish with whole cereals and varied vegetables according to taste and possibilities, observe only the structure, see chapter 7.2)

- Grilled turkey slice with nishime vegetables and pearl barley, pressed lettuce and white radish, spoonful of fermented vegetables
- Boiled millet and tempeh (or meat, fish) on a bed of spinach, pressed salad, a spoonful of fermented vegetables
- Lentil curry with rice, lettuce leaf, spoonful of fermented vegetables, pressed Beijing cabbage

60 min before dinner: big glass of hot water

30 min before dinner: Freshly squeezed juice:

- 1 carrot, 1 stalk of celery stalks, a slice of ginger

- ½ smaller beets, 1 stalk of celery stalks, green coriander

- 1 carrot, ½ smaller beets, slice of ginger

- + in the spring we can add bear garlic or a spoonful of sprouts such as mungo to the juicer.

Snack (if needed):

- You can buy activated/sprouted nuts with a smart flavor here

- Short stewed apple with seeds or plums with poppy seeds

- Goat kefir with unroasted (raw) cocoa or matcha tea powder

- Spicy sprouted chickpeas

- Alternatively, fermented buckwheat bread with lentil spread and kohlrabi

- The rest of lunch (so you know if you're really hungry or just hungry)

- Apple gingerbread

- LC pumpkin cake (low carb variant of snack)

Dinner - soup:

- A mug of broth made of meat bones, if you've been left in the fridge since the last long-drawn broth

- Vegetable soup with miso paste

Dinner - main course:

- Cod baked with carrots and garlic, buckwheat, pressed Beijing cabbage

- Quick vegetables with adzuki beans (or meat)

- Salmon with nishime vegetables and quinoa and pressed lunch salad and a spoonful of fermented vegetable

Tricks to handle it all with ease:

- Plan the cooking of long-drawn broth from meat bones (preferably farm or organic breeding) for the weekend or let it cook on a low flame (pull) overnight. Then use a cup of therapeutic broth before each main meal, or you can use the next day for a quick dinner in the form of a rich pho soup.
- When cooking cereals or legumes, always cook more of them and store them in the fridge so that you can use them the next day, while having a completely different meal.
- Either way, when you cook cereals, cook more of them and the next morning you can cook them with vegetable milk in breakfast porridge.

- **Simple soups with miso paste are very fast**, you can cut vegetables in advance into a lockable box. I use a slicer for very thin slices, so the vegetables are cooked within 5 minutes. If you clean the vegetables under water with a brush, you don't have to scratch them. By alternating different types of vegetables, you can have a completely different soup from the vegetable alkaline broth (see Recipes) every day.

- If you want a richer soup, just pour already cooked legumes, tempeh, natto and various types of cereals into the refrigerator and have a hundred times different soup.

What care you give yourself in your diet and life this way you will feel. Inner satisfaction is something what nobody and nothing can give us.

With love, Nicole

10. SUPPORTING RECIPES

Recipe explanations:

A-I   the food has an anti-inflammatory effect

Marking and calibration:

1 cup = 250 ml

125 cup = 125 ml

¼ cup = 60 ml cup

1 tablespoon = 15 ml

7,5 spoon = 7.5 ml

1 teaspoon = 5 ml

½ teaspoon = 2.5 ml

¼ teaspoon = 1.25 ml

Vegetable alkaline broth
5 min preparation, 15 min and more cooking

Vegetable broth is essential especially for its alkaline effect. In addition to great taste, it contains a large amount of minerals and vitamins. If you are tired, without energy, chills or otherwise weakened, add more root part of the sweet vegetable to the broth. If, on the other hand, you need more relaxing energy, you feel withdrawn and you feel more warm, include more of the green leafy vegetables. The broth is great as the basis of all soups and we can also use it to prepare meals.

We can use residues and slices of vegetables, brooms, tops of root vegetables and leaves, pumpkin seeds or even "waste" (fiber) from the pressing of vegetable juices.

1. Put all vegetables and algae in a pot with **COLD WATER.**
2. **WE DO NOT SALT** (we never salt the broth so that minerals can be released into it; therefore we salt only the final food that we prepare from the broth).
3. We cook for at least 10-15 minutes. In winter, up to an hour for the broth to gain more yang (strengthening) energy.
4. After cooking, drain. We uncompromisingly throw away the boiled vegetables. We can either use the broth straight away or pour it into glasses, let it cool down and store it closed in a refrigerator for up to three days. We can use boiled algae even further in a dish.

We use all tops from carrots, parsley, kohlrabi, celery, all cherries and any vegetables that are already withered, but are not spoiled or moldy.

Vegetable broth acquires a great taste when we use it to use the hollowed out center of the pumpkin (fiber and seeds), which is usually thrown away if it is not dried. We can also use all wild herbs (ivy, nettle, daisy, etc.) and their roots (dandelion or burdock root). If we have our own vegetables or if we buy organic quality, we can boil all the slices and skins from the washed vegetables into the broth without any worries.

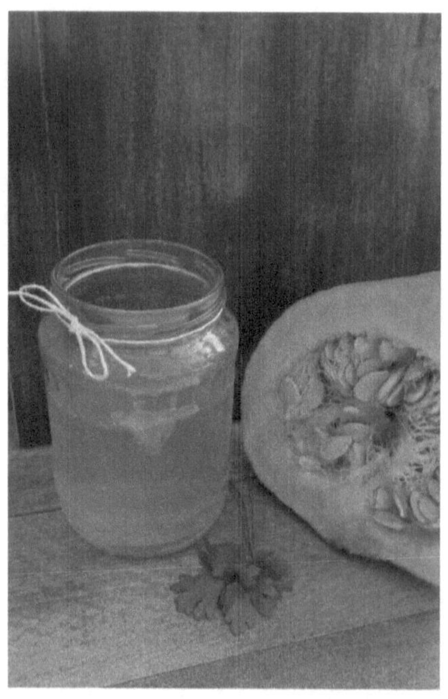

Meat bone broth
5 min preparation, *12 - 24 h cooking*

Strengthens immunity. It strengthens digestion, replenishes energy, nourishes the blood, regenerates, reduces exhaustion, supports the adrenal glands and the energy area of the kidneys. It is an integral part of the treatment of the syndrome of increased intestinal permeability (leaky gut), adrenal exhaustion and the resulting hormonal imbalance.

---

1 kg of beef bones or chicken skeleton, preferably in organic quality
1 onion, 1 carrot 1 parsley
½ celery roots
5 balls of new spices
10 balls of black pepper
2 bay leaves
(in winter we can add a piece of ginger or chili pepper)
5 slices of dried astragalus root

1. (Not absolutely necessary) Bring the water in the pot to a boil and put the bones in it for 3 minutes. This flushes out excess protein. We pour water.
2. Pour a sufficient amount of cold water on the bones; part will boil it, so give it enough. Put the onion in the pot (we can peel only the top skin, so the broth gets a brown color), spices, astragalus and vegetables (we can also put this until the final soup). We can only clean the vegetables with a brush and we don't have to peel them anymore.

3. Bring to a boil and gradually collect the foam over the surface of the soup with a sieve.
4. As soon as the soup starts to boil, we reduce the fire so that it only stretches slightly. We close the lid and we can go to sleep in peace if we have given enough water.
5. We cook 24 hours a day, but of course we can do less. The longer we cook the bones slowly, the more energy/qi we get from them. The bones should really crumble at the end of cooking.
6. Drain the soup and discard the contents of the sieve. Let the broth cool completely so that we can scrape off the excess fat from the surface.
7. Store the broth in the refrigerator for 3-5 days. Therapeutically, we use a cup of warm broth before each main meal or we prepare it with fresh vegetables as a quick morning soup.

I usually cook the broth in the evening and cook it during the day. The soup smells nice and at any time everyone can have a warm cup of broth already during cooking.

Astragalus is a powerful antioxidant, supports physical and mental performance, increases immunity and slows down aging, and is an excellent remedy for all viral diseases.

- has a positive effect on digestion and excretion,
- supports the immune system similar to echinacea,
- detoxifies and reduces inflammation,
- compares blood pressure,
- slows down cell aging,
- reduces the problems associated with premenstrual syndrome and menopause.

Winter strengthening bowl
1 portion, 10 min

Fast, energetically strengthening and rich soup. It warms the digestion and energetically strengthens the center. It also energetically supports the kidneys = the seat of our life energy. If you do not save vegetables, you will significantly reduce the acid-forming tendencies of this breakfast dish. From the point of view of macronutrients, it supplies enough protein, ensures a low glycemic index and saturates. It supports the treatment of the so-called "leaky gut" syndrome, which is one of the causes of many autoimmune diseases.

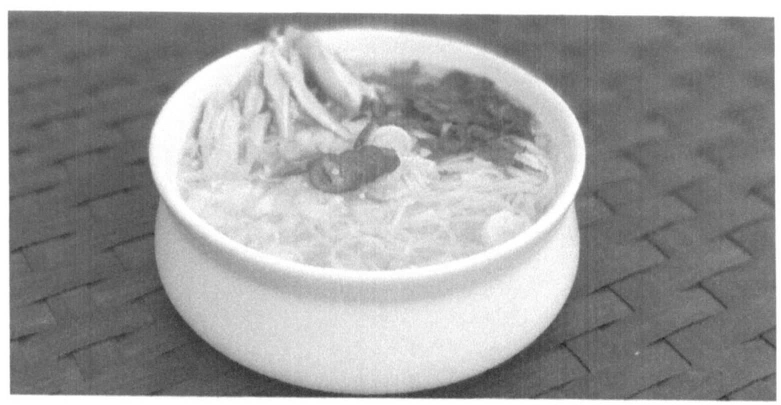

Meat bone broth
Pieces of cooked meat (not necessary)
Leek or spring onion (or any other vegetable) A-I
Rice noodles

(In winter we can add ginger juice A-I or chili pepper A-I)

Steps:

1. Leave thin rice noodles for a few hours, preferably overnight, soaked in a bowl of cold water.

2. Heat the broth and put the drained noodles and finely chopped onion or vegetables in it.

3. Cook briefly so that the noodles and vegetables remain al dente.

4. Serve with a sliced green portion of leek, onion or coriander or chives. Add sprouts in the spring.

Tip: Instead of noodles, you can add the rest of the cooked cereal from the previous day or boil the fermented oat flakes.

Rice porridge with sweet vegetables
1 portion, preparation 5 min, 10 min cooking time

Strengthens digestion. It has a naturally sweet taste. It contains Omega 3 acids and a large amount of fiber. The recipe and ingredients may seem very simple, but they are very harmonizing in the area of digestion. If you take the time and enjoy breakfast, you will feel very well in balance.

1 cup cooked rice
1 cup water
½ tablespoons of flaxseed
½ tablespoons olive oil
1 carrot A-I
4 cm white radish A-I
1 white onion A-I
leaf pack choi or a piece of cabbage A-I
salt

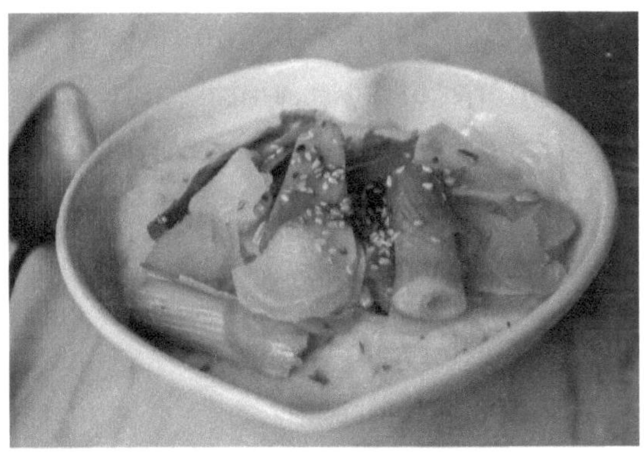

Steps:

1. In a high-bottomed pot, heat the oil and add finely grated carrots and radishes, mix the salt and add about 2 cm of warm water. Place the cabbage on top and cover with a lid. Steam for about 10 minutes (you may need more water, at the end of cooking there should be only a small amount of water left, which is suitable to drink or use).

2. Meanwhile, add water to the rice pot and bring to a boil. You can serve the porridge as follows or mix it with a stick mixer.

3. Rinse the flaxseed, fry dry in a pan, crush or grind in a coffee grinder.

Tips:

If you are going to cook a porridge of uncooked rice, cook straight with the flaxseed, and then mix it with a stick mixer.

To strengthen the immunity, add **the ground kuzu root** and prepare glazed vegetables in an instant. Mix a teaspoon of kuzu in a glass with a small amount of cold water and pour into a pan with the almost finished vegetables. With boiling, the vegetables glaze quickly. The goal is not a culinary experience, but **enrichment with another medicinal food - kuzu**, which:

- strengthens immunity,
- supports digestion,
- and strengthens mental well-being.

Sparse vegetable soup with miso paste
1 portion, 3 min preparation, 5 min cooking time

In addition to enhancing the quality of digestion, this soup also has strong cleansing effects. The shitake sponge is a recognized natural remedy against the so-called civilization diseases. It has **immunostimulatory, antitumor and anti-infective effects**. *It cleanses the blood, is suitable for acne, helps to remove internal tension and improves the energy of the liver. The soup is easily digestible and supports the center of the body (stomach, spleen).*

Ingredients:

3 dried shiitake mushrooms
50 g hokkaido pumpkin A-I
1 carrot A-I
green onion A-I
1 teaspoon (or less, to taste)
shiro miso paste
1 cm algae wakame A-I
salt
water or vegetable broth

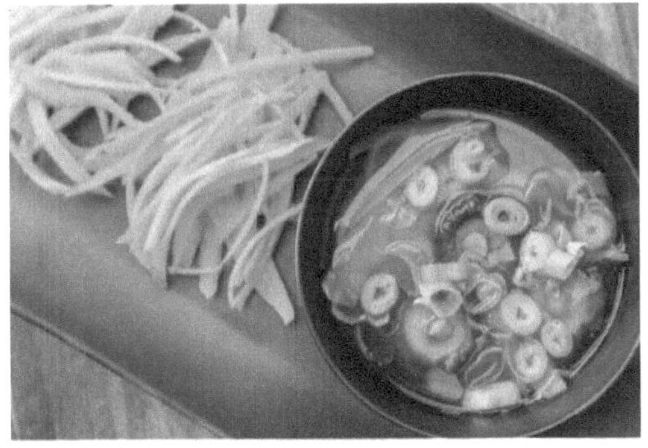

Steps:

1. In the evening or at least 30 minutes in advance, soak mushrooms and algae in a small amount of water (if it was not already part of the broth).
2. Heat the broth or water, including soaking water with shiitake, cut carrots and a piece of hokkaido into matches. (I use a julienne

peeler, which forms straight vegetables on the noodles. The strips are quickly grated, thin, and therefore quickly cooked.)

3. Remove the flame, mix the miso paste in the soup collector and return to the pot. Let stand for 2 minutes and serve garnished with spring onion or other green sprinkles (chives, parsley, coriander, green part of leek).

My tips: Be playful and variable. Rotate the vegetables freely. Try new vegetables that you don't normally eat or that are currently in the fridge or in the garden.

Prepare very quickly, every day, a completely different soup, 2-3 types of vegetables are enough (eg one root and one top).

Congee porridge with gomasio
1 portion, 3 min preparation, 1 – 2h cooking time

Congee porridge is suitable for therapeutic reasons, for chronic or acute digestive problems, general convalescence or cleansing days. This rice porridge is boiled over a low flame for several hours to form a broth. The porridge is easily digestible and strengthens impaired digestion.

You can add crushed **Ashwagandha root** to the porridge during cooking - Ayurvedic herbs that support **physical and mental condition**. Its adaptogenic effects are broad-spectrum. In addition to stimulating effects, it has **antiviral, antibacterial and anti-inflammatory effects**. It also has an aphrodisiac effect.

- strengthens immunity
- reduces stress, anxiety and strengthens concentration
- promotes hormonal balance, fertility, libido and potency
- slows down cell aging

Ingredients:

½ **a cup of rice** (choose the type according to the current condition and weather - brown rice cleanses the intestines and supplies minerals, round-grained has a warm nature, long-grained slightly cooling)

3-5 cups of water
2 cm wakame seaweed
Celtic sea salt or other

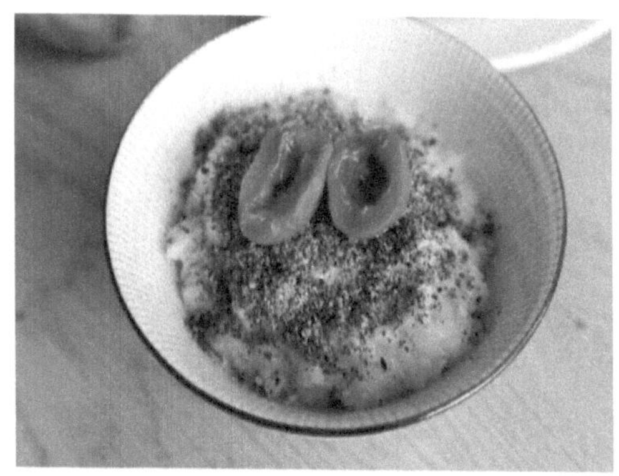

Steps:

Wash the rice well and cook it together with salt and seaweed. Cook over low heat to the consistency of a mash.

How to prepare gomasio:

(roasted black sesame with salt):

1. Fry 1 teaspoon of salt dry in a heavy pan. Roast on medium heat until shiny. We move it aside from the pan.

2. Rinse 12-16 teaspoons of seeds briefly and place on a hot pan. Roast on a medium flame with occasional stirring with a wide wooden spoon and shaking the pan. Once they start to crack softly and smell hazelnut, it's done.

3. Transfer the seeds with salt to a coffee grinder (if you have a mortar, boldly do it) and grind to about 70 %.

4. Let's decorate the porridge. Spread the rest on a plate to keep the gomasio cool, then transfer to a sealable glass and consume soon.

Tip:

You can also boil the remaining seeds of umeboshi plums in the porridge (see chapter 7.4), which will support the acid-base balance, as the rice itself has a slightly acid-forming effect.

Lentil curry with rice

1 portion, 10 min preparation, 45 min cooking time

Ingredients:

0.5 cup red lentils

1.5 cups water / broth

Hokkaido A-I

1 carrot A-I

Cabbage A-I

1 onion A-I

2 cloves garlic A-I

Yellow curry spice A-I

salt, pepper A-I

Ume vinegar

Rice

1 tablespoon hatomugi (not necessary)

Oil

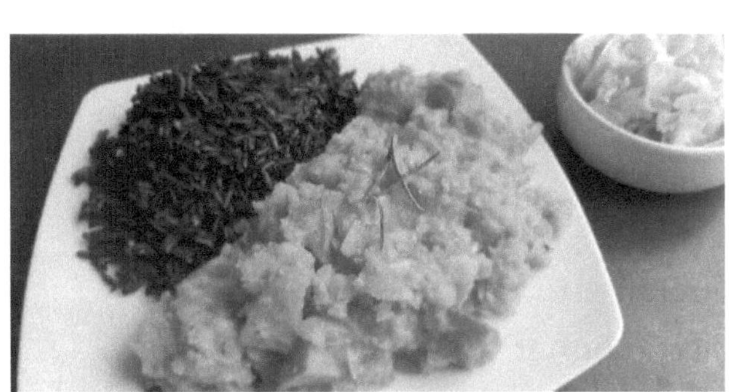

Steps:

1. Boil the rice with pre-soaked hatomugi in twice the amount of water, cook under the lid for 45 minutes.
2. Cut the vegetables into cubes.
3. Heat the oil and fry the onion. Add spices and vegetables in addition to cabbage. We're roasting.
4. Add rinsed lentils and water / broth. Stew 15 min.
5. Finally, mix in the pressed garlic and cabbage.
6. Season with umeboshi vinegar.

Pike perch on baked vegetables
2 portions, 10 min preparation, 20–30 min bake time

2 servings of perch
Mug of rice
1 large carrot A-I
1 parsley A-I
¼ celery A-I
1 onion A-I
Slice of butter
½ tablespoons of oil
Salt pepper
(1 tablespoon alcohol to pour under – not necessary)
200ml vegetable broth or water

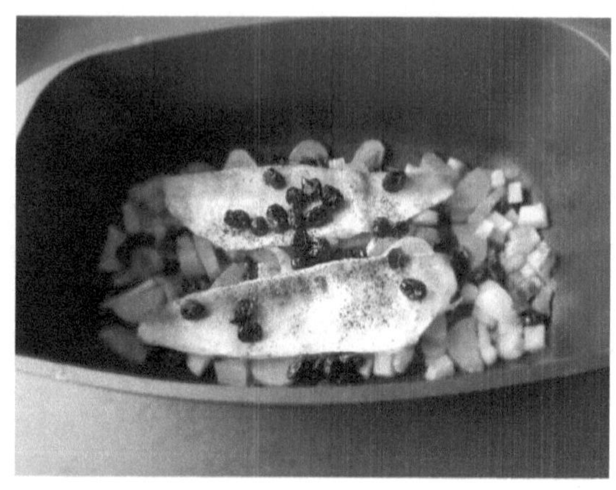

Steps:

1. Preheat the oven to 180 °C.
2. Meanwhile, rub the fillets with oil, salt and pepper; let marinate for a while. Cut the vegetables into half slices, the onion into quarters. Wipe the baking dish with butter, layer the vegetables, add salt and place the fish on top; put uncovered in the oven (or you can spray with alcohol).
3. Let the pre-soaked rice cook.
4. After about 5 minutes, cover the vegetables with hot broth or hot water; cover with a lid and bake until the vegetables are softened, if necessary, pour over.

Natto with rice and compressed salad
2 portions, 10 min preparation, 20 min cooking time

Natto are fermented soybeans** that we buy in most stores with healthy foods. Natto is reminiscent of the socks of a very old homeless man. However, this not very attractive fact is surpassed by the resulting harmonization of blood, which can be perceived even through emotional mental harmony. Personally, after eating natto I feel similar to after meditation. **Natto is a great source of vitamin K2, which is important, among other things, for the transport of calcium to bones and joints.

Ingredients:

Natural rice

Spring onion A-I

A box of natto soybeans

1 teaspoon Shoyu soy sauce

1 teaspoon mustard without preservatives

1 stone from umeboshi plum A-I

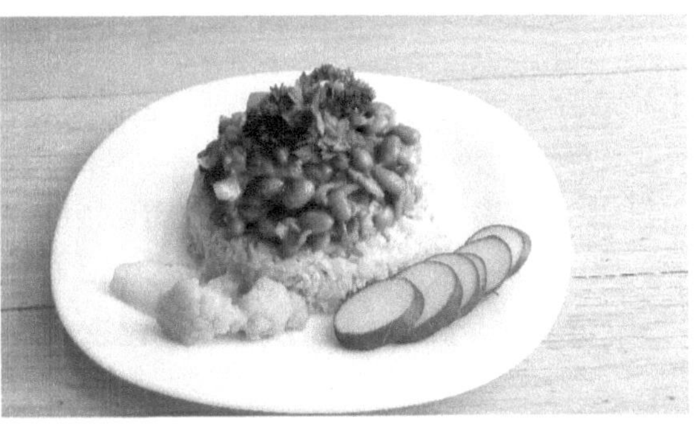

Kombu seaweed 1 cm

Hokkaido pumpkin A-I

Leek A-I

Salt

Ingredients for compressed salad:

Chinese cabbage A-I

Radish A-I
Arugula A-I
Umeboshi vinegar A-I

Steps:

1. Cook the rice together with the stone from umeboshi plum in a pressure cooker for 35 min.

2. Place Kombu seaweed on the bottom of the second pot, layer obliquely chopped leeks on it, layer larger pumpkin cubes on this layer and pour over 1 cm of water, lightly salt and cook under the lid for 12–15 min.

3. Whip the mixture with a teaspoon of soy sauce and mustard in a bowl, mix a spring onion and a box of natto beans into it.

4. Cut cabbage, radish and arugula into fine strips, add a spoonful of umeboshi vinegar, crease and leave for about 30 minutes loaded under a plate, garnish with slightly roasted sunflower seeds.

Tip:

The rest of the soybeans, which we do not process, can be dried on baking paper outside in the sun and added to soups or ground dried beans and used in any dish to enhance the taste. (I don't really recommend drying at home for abrasions, which may not be pleasant. So, better to consume fresh in the winter.

Trout with nishime vegetables
1 portion, 5 min preparation, 25 min bake time

Trout
100 g of white leek
100 g broccoli A-I
1 medium carrot A-I
2 wedges of celery
root A-I
Radish A-I
1 Tbs olive oil
1 Tbs breading from
peas and corn (or any gluten free)
Salt
Umeboshi vinegar A-I
Green parsley A-I
1 cm seaweed

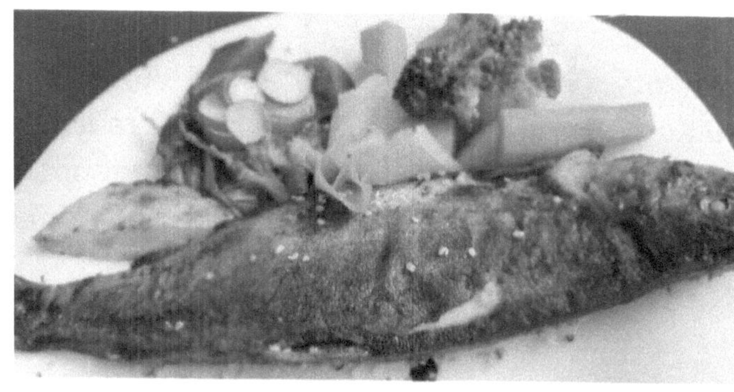

Steps:

1. Preheat the oven to 180 °C. Salt the trout, stuff with green parsley and dry wrap in breading; put in a greased baking dish together with celery and bake in the oven for about 25 minutes.

2. Meanwhile, cut the radishes into thin wheels, drizzle with vinegar and load with a plate.

3. Then we prepare **nishime vegetables**. Put about 1 cm of water in the pot, put algae on the bottom and cook. Cut carrots and leeks diagonally into larger blocks (3 cm), divide the broccoli into roses and put in a pot; cover with a lid.

Cod baked with carrots
1 portion, 10 min preparation, 20 min bake time

Ingredients:
1 serving of cod or any fish
2 carrots A-I
1 onion A-I
1 tablespoon olive oil
Salt, garlic A-I

Rosemary A-I
A piece of cabbage A-I
Arugula A-I
2 radishes
Umeboshi vinegar A-I
Spoon of sunflower and flax seeds A-I

Steps:

1. Preheat the oven to 180 °C. Salt the cod.
2. Cut the cabbage, radish and arugula into fine strips, add a spoonful of umeboshi vinegar, crease and leave loaded under a plate for about 30 minutes.
3. Wrap the cod together with the carrots cut and onion into circles, mixed with pressed garlic, rosemary and a slice of butter in baking paper and bake for about 20 minutes in the oven.
4. Rinse a tablespoon of sunflower and flax seeds briefly in a sieve and transfer to a hot, dry, high-bottomed pan, stirring with a wooden spoon until crispy. Sprinkle the seeds with fish and vegetables.

Fast vegetables with adzuki
2 portions, 10 min preparation, 15 min cooking time

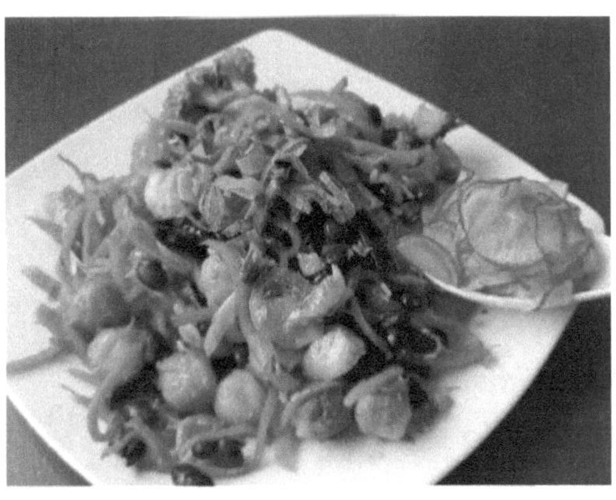

a handful of cooked adzuki beans
1/2 tablespoon coconut oil
1 onion A-I
200g cauliflower A-I
100g mushrooms
Vegetable broth / bean broth
Natural rice
White radish / turnip A-I
Umeboshi vinegar A-I
Red curry paste on the tip of a knife
1 teaspoon red pepper
Salt

Steps:

1. Let the rinsed salted rice cook.

2. Fry the diced onion in a fat pot, add the sliced mushrooms in a chopper, salt and stew.

3. Then add cauliflower, curry, paprika and pepper and pour hot broth. Stew for 10 minutes or until moderate.

4. In the meantime, cut white radish or turnip into thin slices, drizzle vinegar, mix and load.

5. Add beans to the pot with the mixture. We let the tastes connect and we can serve.

6. Garnish with parsley or sprouts. Serve with white radish.

Meat, fish or tempeh with nihime vegetables
1 portion, 5 min preparation, 10 - 15 min cooking time

Nishime vegetables are chopped vegetables, cooked in their own juice, or in a minimal amount of water, with a pinch of salt and seaweed, or a slice of ginger (in winter).

Meat, fish or tempeh
Hokkaido A-I
Parsnip A-I
Leek A-I
Carrots A-I
Broccoli A-I
Algae kombu
Slice of ginger A-I

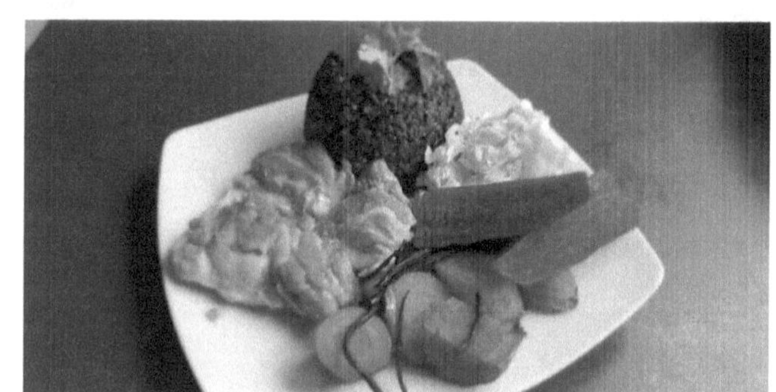

1. Put a slice of algae and ginger on the bottom of the pot, pour about 2 cm of water; for that, we stack the chopped vegetables in addition to broccoli.

2. Cook under the lid for about 10 minutes. Finally, we add broccoli roses. We can drizzle with soy sauce.

3. In the meantime, prepare a slice of meat, fish or marinated tempeh for the contact grill.

4. Serve with whole cereals (rice, quinoa, millet, buckwheat) or only with vegetables in the case of a low-carbohydrate diet.

Apple gingerbread

Size 20 x 20 cm, 10 min preparation, 30 min bake time

Ingredients:

250g of apples A-I

150g of spelled or gluten - free flour

80g of apple concentrate or other sweetener

45g of coconut oil

1 egg

4 tablespoons cocoa

1teaspoon phosphate-free baking powder

1 teaspoon cinnamon A-I

½ teaspoons of ground ginger A-I

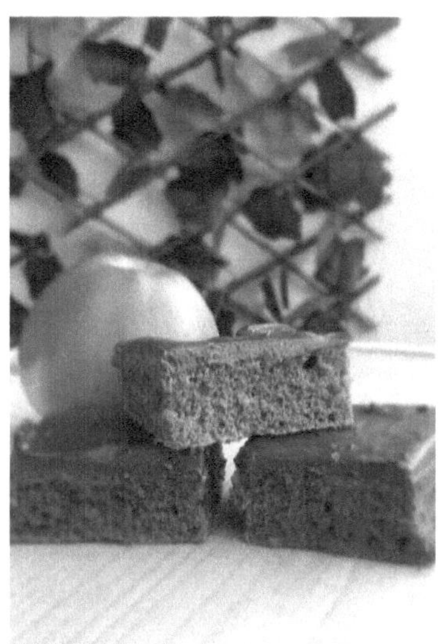

For ganache:

120 g 80% chocolate

200 ml coconut whipped cream

Steps:

1. Heat the oven to 170 °C.
2. Grate the apples, including the skin, or mix smoothly.
3. Add all the ingredients and mix.
4. Bake at 170 °C for about 30 minutes.

Chocolate topping:

Heat the whipped cream so that it does not boil and remove it from the fire. Pour pieces of chocolate into the hot cream and stir with a whisk until the chocolate is completely dissolved. Allow the ganache to partially cool, stirring occasionally, and pour over the cooled dessert.

Low carb pumpkin cake

Size 20 x 20 cm, 10 min preparation, 40 min bake time (without puree preparation)

Ingredients:

320 g pumpkin puree
190 g almond flour
3 happy eggs
90 ml of coconut oil
90 g sweetener (xylitol, erythritol)
90 g of cream cheese
A handful of chopped walnuts
3 teaspoons of phosphate-free baking powder
2 teaspoons gingerbread spices
Pinch of salt

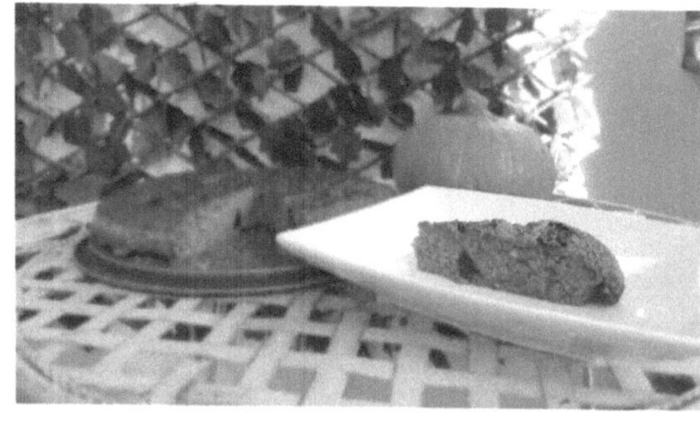

Steps:

1. Prepare pumpkin puree: make a fibrous pulp from the hokkaido pumpkin (from which we cook vegetable broth for soups), cut the pulp into strips, spread on baking paper and bake in the oven for about 20 minutes at 180 °C - I prepare puree for example during baking bread or meat).
2. Put chilled roasted pumpkin in a blender and mix.
3. Add all other ingredients (except nuts and chocolate) and mix until smooth.
4. Mix the nuts into the dough and move to the cleared mold. Push fragments of chocolate into the dough and bake at 170 ° C for about 40 minutes. Allow the cake to cool completely before slicing.

Sprouted chickpeas
90 min (without soaking and germination)

This snack not only satisfies the taste buds, but is also a good source of protein. If you plan its preparation even more and germinate chickpeas, it will be even more valuable. After soaking, just let it germinate for 24 hours (it will create about 2 mm sprouts), so we:
1. *reduced the content of antinutritional substances*
2. *improved digestibility*
3. *increased the content of valuable substances.*

Ingrediets:

100 g of chickpeas

1 tablespoon olive oil

1 teaspoon of spices to taste (Thai spices with turmeric A-I, barbecue spices, garlic A-I, gourmet yeast or smoked paprika)

Sea salt

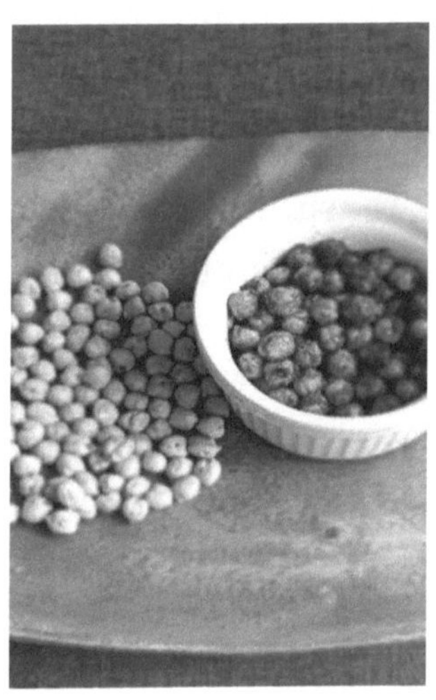

Steps:

1. Soak the chickpeas in water with a spoonful of natural (eg apple cider vinegar) for 12 hours.

(2.) Then rinse and transfer to a germinating container or to any container suitable for germination; eg strainer bowl for spaghetti and cover with a lid. Let it germinate (it is enough if it creates about 2 mm sprouts). Rinse the chickpeas regularly after 12 hours.

Of course, we can also skip this 2nd point and just cook the chickpeas. However, by germination we only get it for our digestion.

3. Rinse the chickpeas and **cook without salt**. Drain the chickpeas and dry in a cloth.

4. Then mix the chickpeas with oil and salt and transfer to baking paper.

5. Bake at 180 °C for about 35 minutes and mix twice in the meantime.

6. Mix the roasted chickpeas with the spices and serve.

Tip:

We always cook legumes without salt. You can also add kombu algae (1 cm) to cook chickpeas, which you can then use later, for example, in a soup.

Fermented buckwheat bread
24 h fermentation, 90 min baking

Although buckwheat is naturally a gluten-free pseudo-cereal, the fermentation process always pays off in terms of better digestibility. Fermentation reduces the content of anti-nutrients and increases the absorption of some minerals. Buckwheat is heating in terms of thermals, which is good to use especially in winter. It is rich in insoluble and soluble fiber, which is an important nutrient for bacteria in the intestinal microflora. In addition to the minerals and vitamins it contains, it is an important routine that supports the flexibility of blood vessels and strengthens their walls.

500 g buckwheat flour
900 ml hot water (up to 40 °C)
2 tablespoons chia seeds A-I
2 tablespoons pumpkin seeds A-I
2 tablespoons sesame seeds A-I
2 tablespoons sunflower seeds A-I
2 tablespoons delicacy yeast
2 teaspoons Celtic salt
2 teaspoons crushed cumin/dry garlic A-I
or spices to taste
coconut oil to clear the mold

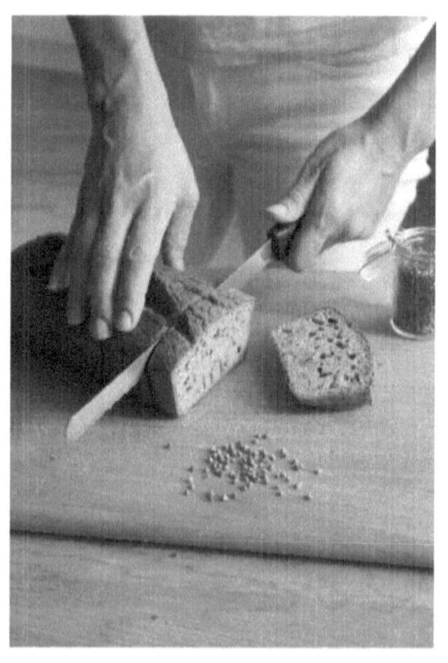

Steps:

1. Mix flour with water, chia seeds and salt in a bowl and mix the dough into a pancake mass to aerate a lot.

2. Cover the bowl with the dough with a cloth and leave to ferment in the heat on the kitchen counter for 24 hours. Sometimes (at least once) we mix so that the dough is more aerated and the microbes can "work". The dough will double its volume by the next day.

3. Mix all other ingredients into the dough (rinse the seeds and fry them dry - we can also use unroasted seeds, but roasting improves their digestibility and they are wonderful in taste. I like to add **black cumin**, it has an onion taste and it is **a natural antibiotic**.

4. Heat the oven to 230 °C together with the already erased mold and carefully transfer the dough to the hot mold and close it with the lid. If we do not have a bread mold with a lid, we can also move the dough into the mold and just put it in an already heated baking dish with a lid.

5. Bake as needed for about 1.5 hours. After baking, carefully tilt the loaf out of the mold and let it cool on the grid.

Fermented cabbage juice

15 min preparation, 60 min under pressure, 3 dny fermentation

---

Fermented cabbage juice is a therapeutic folk medicine supporting the health of the mucous membranes of the intestinal tract, the quality of which is essential for immunity. Helps with digestive problems and infectious diseases. It supports the production of digestive juices and a healthy intestinal microflora. However, if the stomach area is weakened, do not use the juice on an empty stomach, but rather after a meal.

Ingredients:

1 kg red / white cabbage (we can add carrots, onions, beets, a little fresh horseradish, etc.) A-I

1 teaspoon cumin (to taste)

1 teaspoon sea salt

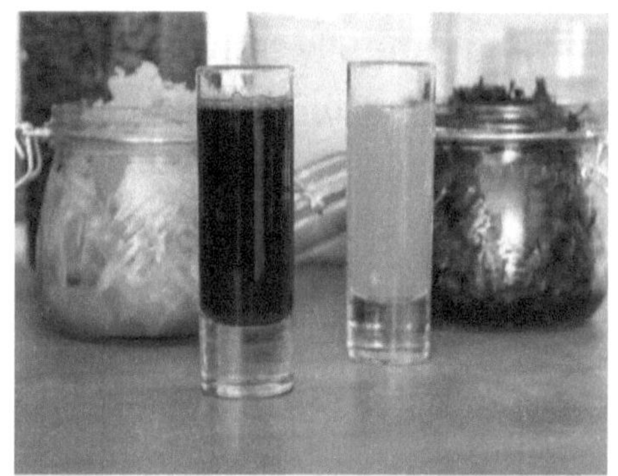

Steps:

1. Finely grate the cabbage and possibly other vegetables. Roughly grate the carrots.
2. Mix everything together, add sea salt, cumin and work well with your hands to break the cell structure and release the juice. You can help by vertical hitting with a meat mallet. Finally, load the cabbage with a plate and a heavy bottle. We leave it loaded for about an hour and thanks to that we release even more juice.

3. Then we start stuffing the vegetables into a glass / container. If you do not have gouache or a glass with a spring, then you must load the vegetables in the container with a plate, a stone or a glass with water.

4. Let the container with the mixture ferment for 3 to 5 days at room temperature. We immediately consume the vegetables or store them in the refrigerator for about 3 months and gradually drink the healthy juice.

Healthy sweet drink
1 portion, 3 min preparation, 20 min cooking time

This medicinal drink is associated with the topic of sweets, uncontrollable tastes, hypoglycemia and insulin resistance. It is naturally sweet. It significantly improves the functioning of the pancreas (with regular drinking) and helps reduce uncontrollable cravings for extreme sweets. You can have it for breakfast during an intermittent fast or at any time during the day. This medicinal drink is a balm for our internal organs and can be drunk every day.

Ingredients:

A piece of hokkaido pumpkin or 1 carrot A-I

1 smaller onion A-I

A piece of cabbage A-I

Steps:

1. Vegetables cut into medium-sized pieces.

2. Add 2 parts of cold (preferably filtered) water to one part of vegetables; bring to a boil and cook for 20 minutes **WITHOUT SALT.**

3. Strain the drink through a plastic sieve and drink warm. We throw away the vegetables, because thanks to the absence of salt, she has already **transferred all her nutrients to this heal drink**.

My tips:

If we lack energy and feel weak, we use 3 types from the following selection of vegetables: hokkaido pumpkin, carrot, parsnip, onion and cabbage.

If we are tense and feel more physical, we prefer white vegetables: white radish - daikon, cabbage, white leek, turnip, and white radish.

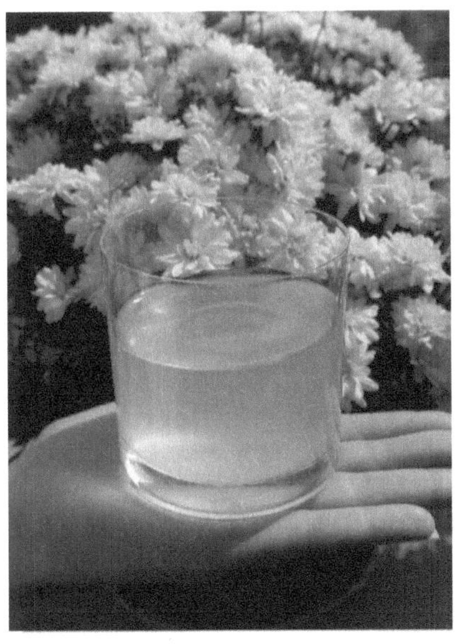

11. CONCLUSION

1. Chew each bite thoroughly.
2. Follow the structure of the plate: 1/2 plate of vegetables (most of which warm, a small portion of fresh and 1 spoon of fermented vegetables), 1/4 plate of meat or legumes, 1/4 plate of side dish.
3. Watch your **anti-inflammatory diet** (ratio of omega 3 and omega 6 and eliminate everything that promotes inflammation - sugar, white bread, trans fats).
4. 30 minutes before the main meal, add consistently salted fresh vegetables or fruits.
5. Eat pickles daily - short-fermented vegetables and other fermented foods.
6. In the morning, include a hot and humid breakfast (soup or porridge), especially on cold days.
7. Of the dairy products, prefer the sour ones.
8. Drink between meals, limit drinking during meals. In the cold season, drink hot drinks. Avoid cold drinks.
9. Don't stress and enjoy life.
10. Go to nature often (barefoot in summer), breathe consciously.
11. Sleep well and sufficiently, i.e. go to bed at 10 pm.
12. Sunbathe daily for 15 minutes from 10-11 am (summer time).
13. **Laugh for 3 minutes a day every day**, whatever, it doesn't matter that it won't be natural, with time it will be. It's about activating and breathing the whole abdominal cavity, and also being in a good mood.

14. Follow this Book and promote digestive quality. Meditate, practice yoga, sleep soundly, enjoy your new lifestyle and approach each other with kindness.

Sources and directions that have influenced me the most:

2009 Chinese Dietetics Course

2009 Workshop The Kushi Institute of Europe

2010 Kurzyatac.cz

2011 Diet according to five elements

2017 Cooking week with MUDr. Vladimira Strnadelova

… And a huge number of books in my library:

Campbell, K. *The WELL-FED microbiome cookbook*. Rockridge Press, 2016.

Fallonová, S. *Nourishing Traditions*. New Trends Publishing, 1999.

Kastner, J. *Chinese Nutrition Therapy*. Georg Thieme Verlag, 2009.

Leggett, D. *Recipes for* Self-Healing. Meridian Press, 1999.

LU,Henry C. *Chinese System of Food Cures*. Sterling Publishing Company, 1986.

Shinya, H. *The Enzyme factor*. Publishers Group, 2010.

Shinya, H. *The Rejuvenation Enzyme*. Ingram International, 2012.

Strnadelová, V., Zerzán, J. The joy of food. ANAG Publishing House, 2011.

Strnadelová, V., Zerzán, J., Joy of healthy children. 3rd edition Olomouc: Nakladatelství ANAG, 2013.

Temeline, B. *The Five-Elements Wellness Plan*. Sterling Publishing Company, 2002.

HOW TO STRENGTHEN IMMUNITY IN 90 DAYS

Learn how to strengthen not only your immunity but also heal your digestion, hormonal, skin and autoimmune diseases with food and proper food preparation!

It will make me happy when you write to me how you manage to increase your immunity thanks to a comprehensive approach in your diet and approach to life, or what health problems have improved in your case.

I appreciate it and thank you for the trust of all those who shared with me how the book moved them in their relationship with themselves.

Send me an email if you missed something in the book or something was too brief. Alternatively, you may want to address your health issues individually.

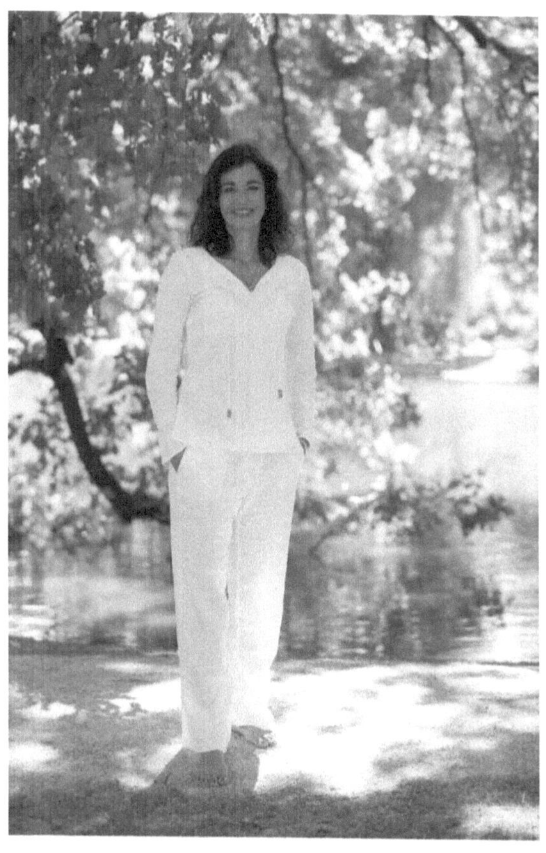

e-mail: jajsem@zdravesnicole.cz

Nicole Lukášková

Holistic health website: www.zdravesnicole.cz

E-shop - Activated (sprouted) nuts with holistic flavor:
www.ziveorechy.cz *"Your snack with inner source of energy"*

FB: https://www.facebook.com/zdravesnicole/

IG: https://www.instagram.com/zdravesnicole/